YOUR HEALTH
AND
YOUR HOUSE

Keats Titles of Related Interest

YOUR HEALTH AND YOUR HOUSE

A RESOURCE GUIDE

Nina Anderson
and Albert Benoist

Keats Publishing, Inc. New Canaan, Connecticut

Your Health and Your House is not intended as medical advice. Its intent is solely informational and educational. Please consult a health professional should the need for one be indicated.

YOUR HEALTH AND YOUR HOUSE

Library of Congress Cataloging-in-Publication Data

Anderson, Nina
  Your health and your house : a resource guide / Nina Anderson and Albert Benoist.
      p.   cm.
  Includes bibliographical references and index.
  ISBN 0-87983-630-X
  1. Housing and health.   2. Sick building syndrome.   3. Consumer education.
I. Benoist, Albert.   II. Title.
RA770.5.A53   1994
613'.5—dc20

94-30819
CIP

Printed in the United States of America

Published by Keats Publishing, Inc.
27 Pine Street (Box 876)
New Canaan, Connecticut 06840-0876

1 3 5 7 8 6 4 2

CONTENTS

HOW TO USE THIS BOOK

YOUR HEALTH AND YOUR HOUSE was designed as a resource guide for anyone suffering from health symptoms that either do not go away or appeared for no apparent reason. Utilization of this book is best approached by:

A. Looking up the symptom in question in the **List of Symptoms and Their Aggravating Pollutants,** Appendix B.
B. Determining from this list which hazards are aggravators.
C. Read the chapter on this hazard and determine if this is a possible cause of the symptom.
D. Determine from the chapters, possible solutions to reducing the symptom.
E. Cross-referencing the aggravator and all othe symptoms it may affect by using the **List of Pollutants and Their Effects,** Appendix C.

FOREWORD

A thoughtful practicing physician will soon perceive that the origins of illness among his patients are often clouded in mystery. It has been estimated that more than 60 percent of office patients suffer symptoms with no definable cause. It is possible that environmental factors may play a role in many of these illnesses.

Patients may present nonspecific symptoms such as fatigue, headache, sore throat, body aches, insomnia and shortness of breath. They present themselves to their doctor, and, strangely, nothing is found wrong. There will be no clues to the cause of the symptoms either in the physical examination or from the usual blood tests.

The problem, up to now, is that although the physician and/ or the patient may suspect some environmental factor, there has been no practical way to confirm or deny these suspicions. This publication, *Your Health and Your House*, is the first comprehensive guide that is available to help you investigate logically whether toxins in the home are responsible for illness.

The authors, Nena Anderson and Albert Benoist, have compiled in one place a remarkable collection of references dealing with toxic effects of substances commonly found in the home. Arranged in a fashion that makes identification possible, these potential toxins are clearly named and tabulated. Evidence is presented to verify the toxicity of various pollutants. Much controversy surrounds the validity of some of these allegations, but the evidence is weighed and an appropriate course of action can be determined. Anecdotal and scientific evidence is presented for consideration. References are abundant, so that more intensive reading is possible.

Classifications are cross-indexed so one can track down the possible toxin either by knowing the symptoms or by knowing the route of entry of the possible toxin. The authors have been thorough, and the guide reflects their industry and understanding. So extensive is their research, that it is somewhat terrifying to learn of so many possible dangers. To avoid the apprehensions of medical students who suffer in turn each illness they learn about, the reader is urged to read with some degree of questioning.

My congratulations are extended to Nena Anderson and Albert Benoist for their fine work.

Harold Gabel, M.D.

YOUR HEALTH
AND
YOUR HOUSE

PREFACE

ACCORDING TO THE Environmental Protection Agency (EPA), 11,400 people will be killed this year by indoor air pollution. Will you be one of them?

Most of the symptoms listed in this book could be explained by a standard medical diagnosis and be treated by normal medical methods. As common characteristics, these symptoms could be the result of initial under- or overactivity of neural, hormonal and enzymatic mechanisms in any target tissue, depending on a patient's susceptibility. This could then be followed by exhaustion of the compensating mechanisms and the development of overt disease. A common cause could be the presence of foreign chemicals competing with natural substances for the same receptor sites in cell walls or enzymes.

Since 1940 we have been exposed to an ever-increasing number of chemicals in our air, food and water. There is no natural evolutionary mechanism in place to eliminate these toxins. The chemicals wind up in our body tissues (see Appendix A). We must become educated if we are to prevent these foreign attackers from entering our bodies and doing their damage.

Most of us, including many in the medical profession, are ignorant of the hazards that accompany the conveniences and new materials we have created in the last 30 years. Some of this ignorance is profit-driven—industry fights hard to prevent us from knowing the truth. Other information may be locked up for years in product testing. Some ignorance may just be based on disbelief and some may be attributed to the age old response, "Well, we have to die of something."

Modern civilization has put convenience first and regard for health second, but with an ever-growing number of unexplainable symptoms arising, people are starting to ask questions. Over 4 million new chemicals have been created since 1915—the effects of four out of five have not been studied on humans. Cancer looms over our heads, along with heart problems, increased cases of asthma, sudden infant death syndrome and AIDS. Epidemiologic studies have implicated the indoor environment as a primary factor in the high prevalence of asthma in New York City.

Could these chemicals that surround us, especially those within our indoor environment, be causing problems or at least aggravating existing ones? We are now discovering the health hazards of combining drugs. Can mixtures of chemicals also cause harmful reactions that affect our health?

Some statistical information is presented here to prod you to ask questions about your own health and its relation to indoor air and water quality:

• Indoor air quality has been receiving attention since people began to assemble in buildings. Benjamin Franklin noted that, "No common air from without is so unwholesome as the air within a closed room that has been breathed and not changed."

• People used to assume that water was safe to drink. In 1900, 27,000 Americans died of typhoid fever, a disease later determined to be transmitted through the water supply. People also once assumed that outdoor air was safe to breathe. In 1970 the EPA was formed to enforce air pollution control regulations.

• People used to assume that indoor air was safe to breathe. In 1985 the Department of Housing and Urban Development required that warning labels be posted in manufactured houses concerning products that cause indoor air pollution and health problems. The EPA report to Congress, dated August, 1989, found that formaldehyde irritates mucous membranes at levels of 0.1 to 0.2 ppm (parts per million). Individuals sensitized to formaldehyde react allergically at concentrations of less than 0.1 ppm.

• The Consumer Federation of America cites indoor air pollution as a major health problem, responsible for up to 50 percent of all illness in the United States each year. Annual cost: $100 billion in medical expenses and lost work time.

• The EPA found that indoor sources may expose home dwellers to levels of toxic air polluted to ten times that of outdoor air.

• Allergies are increasingly aggravated by contact with indoor air pollutants.

• The Surgeon General pointed out in a 1979 report that "There is virtually no major chronic disease to which environmental factors do not contribute, directly or indirectly."

• The American Medical Association reports a 45 percent higher incidence of respiratory infection among occupants of new buildings than among those in older dwellings.

• The Board on Environmental Studies and Toxicology of the National Research Council, the research branch of the National Academy of Sciences, estimates that 15 percent of the population experiences hypersensitivity to chemicals found in common household products.

This book is not based on original material. It is a compilation of information from experts and authors in the fields of indoor environment, government and medicine. A complete bibliography follows the text. We encourage all readers to enhance their knowledge by using our reference sources. The need for a reference guide to indoor air pollutants, the health symptoms they produce and the conditions they aggravate arose from questions asked in our consulting business. We specialize in "healthy house" inspections that identify potential indoor air pollutants. We educate our clients to the hazards of these pollutants and suggest affordable solutions. In an effort to find answers, we sifted through many volumes of material published by government agencies and written by environmentally concerned authors.

In addition, much information was obtained from the growing number of nontoxic product manufacturers. Each reference source gave pertinent information, but only by reviewing many sources did we get a comprehensive picture.

Since we needed a quick reference guide to satisfy our clients' immediate questions, we went to our computer and effectively

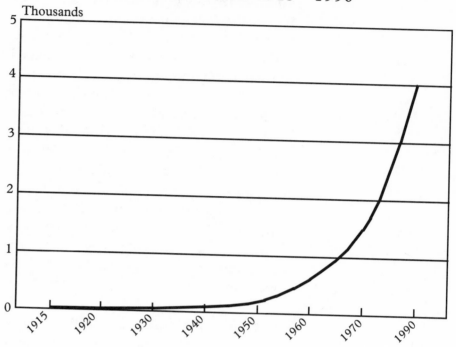

Synthetic Chemicals
Production Rate 1915 - 1990

constructed a database determined by symptoms (see Appendix B), and another database of pollutants with the symptoms they aggravate (see Appendix C). For a list of where to find specific pollutants, see Appendix D.

The supplementary information presented in this book is to be used as a foundation for awareness and further study. It is to be consulted along with any diagnosis or suggested solution to a listed health symptom.

In an effort to be impartial to manufacturers, we hesitate to be more specific in our recommendations for solutions. For a complete listing of these manufacturers of non- or reduced toxicity products, contact Environmental Construction Outfitters, 44 Crosby Street, New York, NY 10012 1-800-238-5008. Canadian readers please contact The Third Loop, 160 Jane Street, Toronto, ONT M65 3Y6. Sales representative Debra Fox (416) 604-4444.

Please note that we do not claim any pollutant to be a cause of any symptom. Any reference to cause is made by the author of the text source. These toxins may aggravate a given condition or contribute to overall health problems in chemically sensitive people over a period of time. We reprint statistics as they appeared in the given sources. Our suggested solutions are not cures, but recommendations for reducing the toxins in the indoor environment. This may not be a comprehensive list, but as awareness grows and new information is presented as to the effects of manmade materials on our health, we will continue to update our database.

CLEAN AIR

THE FOLLOWING CASE findings come from the *Annals of Internal Medicine,* January 15, 1989, published by the Southwest Foundation for Biomedical Research and the University of Texas Health Science Center at San Antonio.

A 60-year-old woman had had recurrent acute migratory pneumonias for nine months. The results of an evaluation, which included tests for serum precipitins, a transbronchial biopsy and a bronchial provocation, confirmed a diagnosis of hypersensitivity pneumonitis caused by an aspergillus species. The findings from gravity air cultures in the home showed a heavy infestation of mold. The installation of electrostatic dust filters in the return ducts of the central air-conditioning system resulted in the lowering of mold colony counts to normal levels. This change in the environment enabled the patient to live at home without having the signs and symptoms of hypersensitivity pneumonitis, or a need for medication.

Thirty months after the electrostatic dust filters were installed, total mold colony counts were still normal, the patient remained free of the signs and symptoms of hypersensitivity pneumonitis and serum precipitins could no longer be demonstrated. Electrostatic dust filters may be an effective treatment for patients with hypersensitivity pneumonitis when avoidance of the causative antigen cannot be easily and rapidly achieved.

CLEANING INDOOR AIR

The purpose of this section is to educate the reader as to the methods currently used to clean and exchange indoor air. The best way, of course, of reducing the effects of indoor air pollutants is to never have installed toxic materials in a building at all. But if they are already in place, the only solution other than removal is to install a heat recovery ventilator to remove polluted air and/or install an air cleaner to capture pollutants.

HEAT RECOVERY VENTILATORS

Adequate ventilation is critical for all types of housing, but the advent of superinsulation has brought the need for a discrete mechanical ventilation system into the spotlight. WIth virtually airtight construction, and high R values (a measurement of insulation ability), low heating bills become a major consideration when deciding whether to purchase a home. The problem comes when the inhabitant has to decide whether to open windows and let the heat out or keep the house closed and trap indoor air pollutants.

All homes have some openings which leak cold air into, or heated air out of, the house. Even when the windows and doors are closed, air can leak in around their frames, around pipes or electrical outlets, or through cracks between the framing and the foundation. The more complicated the house shape, the greater the opportunity for leaks.

To reduce the energy penalty that these leaks cause, energy codes identify areas to seal against air leakage. Once these leaks are sealed and energy efficiency is realized, more air is trapped inside. The air quality of a house also depends on the number and severity of the pollution sources in the house, and how fast the pollutants are being removed, whether by exhaust fan or through air leaks. A tight house can have acceptable indoor air quality if it contains no major pollution sources, and conversely a "leaky" house can have poor air quality if lots of sources are present.

Because the technology is new, and because most building professionals have rarely had to provide a special ventilation system for detached, single-family houses, ventilation and air quality concerns are frequently overlooked. Mechanical ventilation with a properly sized and installed air-to-air heat exchanger is the major option for the ventilation system in superinsulated houses. Needed ventilation can be supplied without action by the occupants and at lower cost than with other strategies, such as opening windows or running exhaust fans.

DEFINITION

An air-to-air heat exchanger is a heat recovery ventilation (HRV) device that pulls stale, warm air from a house and transfers the heat in that air to the fresh, cold air being pulled into the house. Heat exchangers do not produce heat; they only exchange heat from one airstream to the other. Residential heat exchangers come in two basic types: small, through-the-wall units that are about the size of a room air conditioner, and central, ducted, whole-house models, many of which are about the size of a typical water heater. Efficient models can recover as much as 70 to 80 percent of the heat in the stale air. Although available since the 1970's, they have been unavailable for home usage until recently and are now being manufactured by many companies.

STATISTICS

Leak rates are measured as air exchanges per hour. The average house has a leak rate of .5 to 1.5, but this is not a constant rate owing to wind, temperature, seasons and room location. The minimum air exchange rate recommended is .5. Sweden has made 0.5 ach (air changes per hour) a mandatory year-round continuous minimum (continuous exchange demands a mechanical ventilation system). California recently set a 0.7 ach minimum for winter design conditions for areas of the state where superinsulation is used.

Kitchens need an air exchange rate of 7 if gas cooking equipment is in use. In a typical 1,200-square-foot house, a whole-house heat exchanger could provide up to about 1 ach over the house's natural air leakage rate.

The American Society of Heating, Refrigerating and Air Conditioning Engineers (ASHRAE) set standards for minimum ventilation levels of continuous amounts of air entering each room at 10 cubic feet per minute (cfm), 100 cfm in kitchens and 50 cfm in bathrooms. This assumes exhaust fans will be installed in kitchens and bathrooms. Most manufacturers list the capacity of heat recovery ventilators in air exchange by cubic feet per minute. They normally range from 120 to 700 cfm. Assuming an average 8-foot ceiling in a 3,000-square-foot home, you will need a minimum of about 400 cfm to meet a 1.0 ach level. This level can be raised by usage of kitchen and bath exhaust fans.

Formula to determine cfm needed:
Square foot of house × ceiling height divided by 60 = cfm

Heat recovery ventilators are available as retrofits for existing structures. They can either be in the form of a portable model resembling a piece of furniture with the exhaust hose exiting a temporary portal or window modification, or they can be permanent, installed through a wall fixture. These models have lower cfm's and are therefore for smaller buildings—those under 1,200 square feet. Larger structures require whole-house units that must be ducted to air intakes within the home; these units are best for new construction or homes with forced hot air heating. Most heat recovery ventilators have filters to remove outdoor pollutants before they enter a home and to help keep the unit clean.

Heat exchangers may be a cost-effective way to solve difficult excess moisture problems in conventional housing. Some units have humidistats to control indoor humidity levels. In summer, the rejection of outdoor humidity by those units reduces the air-conditioning load; retention of moisture in winter reduces the need for humidification. The solution to excess humidity is not to go back to loosely constructed homes, but to properly manage the indoor air environment.

Cost effectiveness is based on climate, the cost of fan energy consumed, machine efficiency and the fuel cost for heating. Also included is the lifestyle of the occupants and the thermostat levels they set. The cost of the machine and installation are also considered. In a house without a heat exchanger, one is paying 100 percent of the cost of heating air entering by natural means. In a house with a heat exchanger that is 70 percent efficient, one is paying roughly one-third of this cost of heating air for ventilation, plus the cost of fan energy and machine maintenance. Estimates are 25 cents per day for operation. Economics is not always the deciding factor, however. More important are safety, good quality indoor air, comfort, quiet operation and the ability to automatically ensure adequate ventilation. Prices of HRV's range from $575 to $3,500.

> At noon you can still tell what you had for breakfast by the lingering odors. I'm a late worker and a late riser. Usually when I get up in the morning my wife has already fixed breakfast for the children. My son wants his French toast or pancakes "burned." Before installing my HRV (manufactured by E-Z-Vent), I got up to the disgusting smell of burned breakfast. I could even tell which one was burned. Now, approximately one half hour after my children leave for school, I get up to the sweet smell of clean air.
>
> —*Nicholas H. Des Champs, PhD*

Should a house be built tightly? The State of Maine Energy Resources experts agree that the answer to this question is "yes." But many homeowners ask, "If I build my new home tightly, isn't it likely that the indoor air quality will worsen?" The answer is "no" . . . provided you follow these guidelines:

A. Eliminate most of the pollution sources
B. Construct the house properly
C. Install a ventilation system and, if necessary,
D. Clean the air.

DETECTION

Air exchange rates can be tested by professionals using a blower door, a device that pressurizes a house to get an estimation of the air change rate.

SOLUTIONS

HRV Benefits

- Provides good air quality year-round
- Controls when and where outdoor air enters the building
- Distributes fresh air to rooms
- Introduces outdoor air in a way that avoids drafts and preserves comfort
- Saves up to 85 percent in costs to heat and cool outdoor air compared with nonheat recovery ventilation systems
- Removes moisture or cooking odors from bathrooms, kitchens and other "wet" rooms
- Gives an occupant the ability to remove stale air from all habitable rooms
- Avoids energy waste and discomfort from excessive infiltration.

FOR MORE INFORMATION

- "Heat Recovery Ventilation for Housing," Energy Administration Clearinghouse, Michigan Department of Commerce, (517)373-0480
- Energy Hotline: 1-800-292-4704
- Video: "Introduction to Ventilation and Heat Recovery Ventilation," Conservation Energy Systems, Canada 1-800-667-3717, US (306) 242-3663

MANUFACTURERS

Air Exchange (HRV) (617) 871-4816, Rockland, Maine
DEC International (608) 222-3484, Madison, Wisconsin
E-Z Vent (HRV) (703) 291-1111, Natural Bridge Station, Virginia
Fan America (Vent) (813) 359-3616, Sarasota, Florida
Honeywell (HRV) (612) 542-3357, Golden Valley, Minnesota
Nutech (HRV) (519) 457-1904, London, Ontario, Canada
Nutone (513) 527-5112, Cincinnati, Ohio
Titon, Inc. (Window Vent) (219) 271-9699, South Bend, Indiana
VanEE (HRV) 1-800-667-3717, Minneapolis, Minnesota
Vent-Aire (HRV) (719) 599-9080, Colorado Springs, Colorado

AIR FILTRATION

There is no practical way to completely keep airborne dust, tobacco smoke and pollen particles out of your home. All can originate indoors, especially tobacco smoke. In addition, they can drift into homes that are not airtight or can be carried in with normal activity. These particles would settle eventually, but an air cleaner removes them while they are airborne, thus reducing their concentration in the air and preventing their buildup.

Air pollutants fall into two categories: the off-gassing of organic chemicals and pesticides and particulates such as pollen, dust, mold and dander. Air filters can be an integral part of forced hot air heating systems, but they may not be effective in eliminating all indoor pollutants. They are almost always incorporated into heat recovery ventilators, where they have a better removal rate than in furnace systems. To be sure your efforts are being effective, purchase an air filtration device that is suited to the contaminants you wish to remove.

DEFINITION

Air filtration units absorb, capture or dissolve pollutants and can be used in combination for desired effects. Air purifiers employ several different types of filtration.

Activated carbon works by adsorption (particles stick to the carbon). This carbon must be one-inch thick for efficiency, with the most popular media being coconut-shell carbon. Sometimes these filters are impregnated for specific substance removal, such as copper-nickel salt, which adsorbs formaldehyde. Activated carbon filtration is good for cigarette smoke, gases, odors, mildew, formaldehyde and pesticides and has a six-month life, depending on the intensity of the pollution. A double-activated carbon chamber system will also dilute radon.

Potassium permanganate is activated alumina impregnated with potassium. It absorbs and adsorbs gases and destroys them by oxidation. Normally used with activated carbon filters, it is good for formaldehyde, hydrogen sulfide and ethylene. This filter has a six-month life, depending on intensity of pollution, but lasts longer if used with a particulate-type filter.

HEPA (high-efficiency particulate arrestance) filtration was developed by the U.S. Atomic Energy Commission to filter out dangerous small particles. To meet the HEPA standard, the filter media must remove a minimum of 99.99 percent of all particles in the air down to .3 microns in size, and the efficiency must improve with use. At 95 percent efficiency, 165 particles pass through compared with 1 particle at 99.97 percent efficiency. HEPA filters remove mold spores if the humidity level is at 50 percent or less, but if high humidity is present, mold will grow on the filter. They are good for dust, pollen, mold spores and dead insect parts, and also remove lead dust if it becomes airborne. HEPA filters are useful in large heating systems as well as home units and have a one- to two-year life when used with a pre-filter.

Electrostatic precipitators work by attracting particles by electricity, creating a charge that these particles stick to. They attract dust and particles, pesticides, smoke, bacteria and some viruses. They must be cleaned often when efficiency drops, usually because of clogging. If dust remains on these filters, they can get hot (fry) and release toxins. These toxic gases can be inhaled and cause symptoms.

A polycarbonate filter uses a static electric charge to act like an electrostatic precipitator. It also attracts dust and particles and therefore must be cleaned at least once a month (remove and wash). This type of filtration is normally used in conjunction with commercial heating systems.

The negative ion generator is a unit that changes the electrical charge of its surroundings, thereby attracting particles and dust which drop out of the air onto the surface of the floor near the unit. The generator attracts small particles and is especially useful for reducing cigarette smoke and odors. This type of unit must also be cleaned often.

Ozone generators create activated oxygen, which has an extra atom attached to its molecule. That extra atom breaks down certain chemicals and dissipates them, thus releasing the extra atom in the process. It is effective in drawing out gases from surface materials, such as the volatile organic compounds (VOCs) in adhesives used for carpets and countertops. It is also good for mold and odors. Ozone in high doses can have adverse health effects, therefore only devices approved and restricted to safe levels of emission should be used in homes.

STATISTICS

The Austin Health Report states that millions of children get up tired each morning because of asthma and allergies that interfere with a good night's sleep. The long-term effects can be devastating. Many parents have a tendency to ignore what they consider to be a minor problem and end up with children unable to compete. It has been estimated by Dr. Allan Knoght, a leading expert in this field, that 80 percent of asthmatics do not get proper treatment. The best treatment of asthma and allergy is to avoid their causes. Since highly allergenic pollen grains are bigger and heavier than dust or tobacco smoke particles, they do not stay airborne long. With activity or air currents, pollen grains are constantly stirred up, only to settle again. With an air cleaner operating, however, the grains are removed each time they become airborne, so their concentration in a closed room is gradually reduced, helping to free the allergy sufferer from symptoms

For the acutely sensitive and those who are chemically sensitive, a great deal of benefit can be derived from air cleaners.

The Association of Home Appliance Manufacturers established a clean air delivery rate (CADR) for room air cleaners. The number listed on the seal on the back of the unit corresponds to the amount of air (in cubic feet per minute) cleaned of a specific particle. As a general rule, the higher the CADR, the less time it will take to remove the same amount of airborne particles from a same-size room.

Minutes to Achieve 90% Removal of Airborne Particles
(assumes an air cleaner is operating)

CADR	Dust	Smoke	Pollen
25	49	51	17
40	36	37	15
80	21	21	12
150	12	12	8
300	6	6	5

The chart on the next page indicates some of the pollutants that normally are filtered out by air cleaners, heat recovery ventilators equipped with filtration devices and furnace filters. The particulates with values over ten microns can be seen with the naked eye and do not need dense filters. The smaller the value, the denser the filter must be to trap small micron paticulates.

DETECTION

Dust and particulate tests are available from local labs. These can be performed by a technician or dust samples can be mailed in for analysis. Some do-it-yourself gas tests (formaldehyde, carbon monoxide) are available from catalogues and eco-stores.

SOLUTIONS

Install efficient filters on existing heating or air-conditioning whole-house systems, if applicable, and change or clean them as recommended. Purchase air purification units for the specific pollutants or combinations you desire to remove.

Houseplants are nature's air filters; they breathe in carbon dioxide and breathe out oxygen. Some plants thrive on the very chemicals that are poisonous to humans. Dr. Bill Wolverton, who began studying indoor plants for spaceships and space sta-

Air Infiltration Particulates
To determine proper air filtration

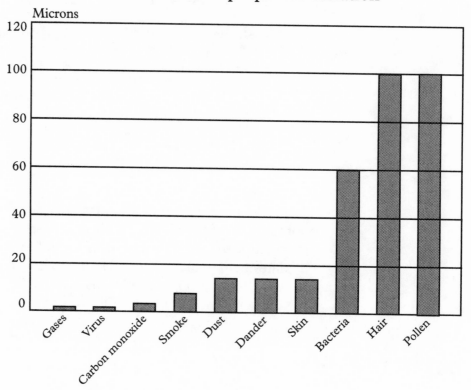

Gases: ammonia, carbon monoxide, formaldehyde, lead, nitrogen oxide, pesticides, sulfur dioxide, phenol, plastic emissions

Virus: mold spores/virus, from .01 to 2 microns

Carbon: particles

Smoke: cooking, wood and tobacco, from .2 to 10 microns

Dust: household and insecticide, from .1 to 15 microns

Dander: animal

Skin: human flakes

Bacteria: from 1 to 80 microns

Hair: human

Pollen: plant

tions at NASA, has improved on nature by creating a carbon-filtered fan-aerated pot which holds a houseplant and increases the plant's air cleaning capacity. Listed below are some common plants and the toxins they remove.

Plant Name	Toxin Removed
Aloe vera	Formaldehyde
Banana	Formaldehyde
Chinese evergreen	Toluene, benzene
Elephant ear philodendron	Formaldehyde
English ivy	Benzene
Ficus	Formaldehyde
Golden pothos	Carbon monoxide, benzene, Formaldehyde
Janet Craig (corn plant)	Benzene
Peace lily	Benzene, trichloroethylene
Spider plant	Carbon monoxide

Wolverton Environmental Services, *Earth Journal*, Nov./Dec., 1993.

FOR MORE INFORMATION

"Consumer Guide for Room Air Cleaners" ($1), Association of Home Appliance Manufacturers, 20 N. Wacker Drive, Chicago, Illinois 60606

MANUFACTURERS

Aireox (714) 689-2781, Riverside, California
AllerMed (214) 422-4898, Wylie, Texas
Austin Air Systems (Aquarius Health) (716) 298-4686
CRSI (317) 839-9135, Plainfield, New Jersey
Dust Free, Inc. 1-800-441-1107, Royse City, Texas
Filtrx (914) 638-9708, New City, New York
Neo Life Company, Fremont, California
Quantum Electronics (401) 732-6770, Warwick, Rhode Island
Thurmond 1-800-AIRPURE, Plano, Texas
Alpine Air (612) 780-9388 Blaing, Minnesota

ASBESTOS

DESCRIPTION

ASBESTOS IS A mineral fiber. It can be positively identified only with a special type of microscope. There are several types of asbestos fibers. In the past asbestos was added to a variety of products to strengthen them and to provide heat insulation and fire resistance.

Most products made since the 1970's do not contain asbestos. Common products that may have contained asbestos in the past include:

1. Steam pipes, boiler and furnace ducts insulated with an asbestos blanket or asbestos paper tape
2. Resilient floor tiles (vinyl asbestos, asphalt and rubber), the backing on vinyl sheet flooring and adhesives used for installing floor tile
3. Cement sheet, millboard and paper used as insulation around furnaces and wood-burning stoves
4. Door gaskets in furnaces, wood stoves and coal stoves
5. Soundproofing or decorative material sprayed on walls and ceilings
6. Patching and joint compounds for walls and ceilings and textured paints
7. Asbestos cement roofing, shingles and siding
8. Artificial ashes and embers sold for use in gas-fired fireplaces
9. Household products such as fireproof gloves, stove-top pads, ironing board covers, hair dryers, automobile brake pads and linings, clutch facings and gaskets.

18

Asbestos exposure can affect almost every organ of the body. Illnesses associated with asbestos are lung cancer, mesothelioma (a cancer of the chest and the abdominal cavity) and asbestosis, in which the lungs become scarred with fibrous tissue. Asbestos-related diseases, sometimes not appearing until 20 to 30 years after contact, can result from very brief exposure and even from contact with people who have been exposed or who may have fibers in their hair or clothing. Most people exposed to small amounts of asbestos, as we all are in our daily lives, do not develop these health problems.

Once inhaled, asbestos fibers lodge in the lungs. Because the material is durable, it persists in tissue and concentrates as repeated exposures occur over time. Most asbestos-related problems are seen in workers who have had prolonged contact with the substance. The health effects of lower exposures in the home are less certain. However, experts are unable to provide assurance that any level of exposure to asbestos fibers is completely safe.

The EPA recommends that if you suspect the presence of asbestos, leave it alone. Most asbestos becomes hazardous as dust is formed when the material is cut or moved.

STATISTICS AND STUDIES

Autopsy reports show that 100 percent of urban dwellers have asbestos in their tissues. This is a frightening statistic since the EPA announced in 1972 that there is no safe level of asbestos exposure. Any exposure to the fibers involves some health risk.

The EPA estimates that there are asbestos-containing materials in most of the nation's approximately 107,000 primary and secondary schools. Properly timed inspections can avoid hazardous situations. Fortunately, most asbestos-containing material can be safely and properly managed in place. Asbestos that is well managed and maintained in good condition appears to pose relatively little risk to building inhabitants and schoolchildren.

Dr. Alfred Zamm, author of *Why Your House May Endanger Your Health*, wrote that he visited a neighbor who had just bought a wood-burning stove: "To protect the wall, he was installing a sheet of asbestos. The dust swirled about his head, and every breath carried minute particles into his lungs. Here was an intelligent man who knew from having read newspapers and magazines of the deadly afflictions that workers in asbestos plants contract from breathing the dust. And here he was permitting this carcinogen in his own home. I was upset with my neighbor and I was upset because the sheet had no cautionary label on it. Such material should have the same warning as iodine bottles, complete with skull and crossbones. Actually, sheet asbestos is more dangerous than iodine, because no adult is going to swallow iodine accidentally; yet my neighbor was breathing asbestos dust."

How many home owners installing a new wood-burning stove protect the wall behind the unit with a sheet of asbestos? This simple but effective method for reducing heat damage could give these home owners health problems later in life. Cutting asbestos spews copious amounts of dust into the air; if the installer does not use a proper face mask, he or she will inhale the toxic substance.

DETECTION

It is important to seek professional advice in identifying potential asbestos problems. If you must handle asbestos in order to obtain a sample for testing, these safety rules should be followed.

A. Make sure no one else is in the room
B. Wear disposable gloves and a dust mask (the type for toxic vapors)
C. Shut down any heating or cooling systems to minimize spread of fibers
D. Place a plastic sheet on the floor below the sample area
E. Wet the material using a fine mist and a few drops of detergent (reduces release of fibers)

   F. Carefully cut a sample and place it into small clean container that has a tight seal

   G. Carefully dispose of the plastic sheet and clean the area with a damp towel; use state procedures for disposal

   H. Patch sample area with duct tape

   I. Send sample to an EPA-approved lab: To get a list of labs, contact the Laboratory Accreditation Administration, Gaithersburg, Maryland 20899, (301) 975-4016.

Note: It is safer to get a licensed asbestos inspector to take samples.

The potential for an asbestos-containing material to release fibers depends primarily on its condition. If the material has become friable—that is, if the material can be crumbled by hand pressure—it is more likely to release fibers, especially when damaged. Any inspection that reveals deteriorating asbestos should be treated as a serious situation. The asbestos should be contained or professionally removed immediately.

SOLUTIONS

Solutions should be suggested by a professional asbestos removal company. If you suspect the presence of asbestos and the product is not cut or damaged and not going to be dislodged during remodeling, leave it alone. Do not use abrasive cleaners on any products suspected of containing asbestos. Do not make even minor repairs to asbestos-containing materials.

When choosing an asbestos removal or repair contractor, contact the EPA's regional office and the Occupational Safety and Health Administration's regional office. They will tell you what regulations the contractor should be following to protect you and the environment from asbestos pollution during the removal or repair.

Good News

Products currently being manufactured that contain asbestos which could be inhaled are required to be labeled. The EPA's

Asbestos Ban and Phaseout Regulation, issued in July, 1989, requires the phaseout of almost all uses of asbestos by 1997.

On October 22, 1986, President Reagan signed AHERA (Asbestos Hazard Emergency Response Act). The act requires the EPA to develop regulations creating a comprehensive framework for addressing asbestos hazards in schools. If financial assistance is needed for remediation, it is comforting to note that since 1985, the EPA has provided over $200 million in loans and grants through the Asbestos School Hazard Abatement Act program. These have helped financially needy public and private schools correct serious asbestos hazards.

Litigation continues over asbestos health issues. According to a report in *The Wall Street Journal*, August 9, 1993, a state court ordered three companies—Westinghouse Electric, Dresser Industries and CSR Ltd.— to pay shipyard workers exposed to asbestos more than $9 million in compensatory damages plus hundreds of millions of dollars of punitive damages.

FOR MORE INFORMATION

- The Toxic Substance Control Act Assistance Information Service Hotline, (202) 554-1404
- Brochures:
  "The ABC's of Asbestos in Schools," EPA, 1-800-368-5888
  "Asbestos (Environmental Backgrounder); The Inside Story—A Guide to Indoor Air Quality," EPA, 401 M Street SW, Washington, DC 20460
  "Asbestos in the Home," EPA, TSCA Assistance Information Service, 401 M Street SW, Washington DC, 20460
  "Indoor Air Pollution Fact Sheet—Asbestos: Air Pollution in Your Home?" American Lung Association
  "Recommended Work Procedures for Resilient Floor Covers," Resilient Floor Covering Institute, 966 Hungerford Drive, Suite 12B, Rockville, Maryland 20850 (enclose stamped/addressed envelope)
- Consumer Products Safety Commission Hotline 1-800-638-8270

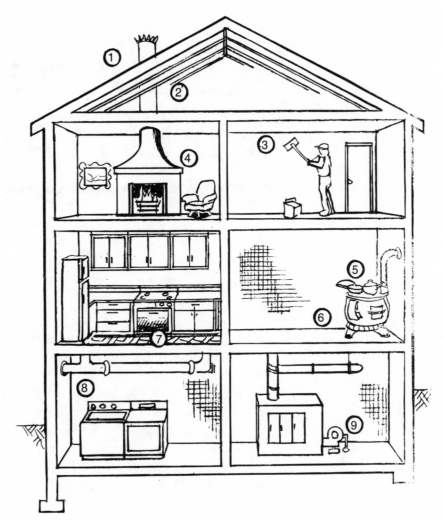

WHERE ASBESTOS HAZARDS MAY BE FOUND IN THE HOME

1. Some roofing and siding shingles are made of asbestos cement.
2. Houses built between 1930 and 1960 may have asbestos as insulation.
3. Asbestos may be present in textured paint and in patching compounds used on wall and ceiling joints. Their use was banned in 1977.
4. Artificial ashes and embers sold for use in gas-fired fireplaces may contain asbestos.
5. Older products such as stove-top pads may have some asbestos compounds.
6. Walls and floors around woodburning stoves may be protected with asbestos paper, millboard or cement sheets.
7. Asbestos is found in some vinyl floor tiles and the backing on vinyl sheet flooring and adhesives.
8. Hot water and steam pipes in older houses may be coated with an asbestos material or covered with an asbestos blanket or tape.
9. Oil and coal furnaces and door gaskets may have asbestos insulation.

COMBUSTION POLLUTANTS

CARBON MONOXIDE, nitrogen dioxide, respirable particles and sulfur dioxide are listed together because they stem from similar sources.

Combustion pollutants are gases or particles that come from burning materials. The common fuels burned in appliances are natural or liquid propane gas, fuel oil, kerosene, wood or coal. The types and amounts of pollutants produced depend on the type of appliance, how well it is installed, maintained and vented and the kind of fuel it uses.

CARBON MONOXIDE

DESCRIPTION

Carbon monoxide (CO) is a colorless, odorless gas that interferes with the delivery of oxygen throughout the body. At low concentrations, it can cause fatigue in healthy people and episodes of increased chest pain in people with chronic heart disease. Carbon monoxide at higher concentrations can cause headaches, dizziness, weakness, nausea, confusion, disorientation and ulti-

24

mately unconsciousness and death. Other side effects include impaired vision and coordination and flulike symptoms that clear up after exposure.

Carbon monoxide poisoning is really asphyxiation from oxygen deprivation. The invisible, odorless gas attaches firmly to hemoglobin, the red pigment of blood; it occupies portions of the molecule normally available to transport oxygen from the lungs to the rest of the body. When 50 to 80 percent of the hemoglobin becomes blocked by carbon monoxide, the brain dies; if the buildup has been rapid, there may be very little warning. If the level rises more slowly, 30 to 50 percent of the hemoglobin may be blocked resulting in little more than flulike symptoms. A more rapid rise to such high levels causes headache, dizziness, confusion and nausea. When the level is at 2 to 4 percent, which is common in everyday situations, the symptoms are relatively subtle, though unpleasant. Impairment of thinking and fine motor coordination has been observed. In the *Harvard Medical School Health Letter* of March, 1990, Vol. 15, No. 5, new research was reported to show that even at "normal" CO contaminant levels, the heart is affected.

The presence of CO can be determined by a blood test that measures the blood level of CO combined with hemoglobin. Because CO leaves the blood slowly, this test can pinpoint a problem even if the blood is drawn one or two hours after one has left a suspected environment.

Carbon monoxide is measured in parts per million (ppm). In today's motor-vehicle-laden industrial world, we can find levels of 15 ppm in residential areas and from 5 to 50 ppm in cars that are being driven. The ambient air around Los Angeles frequently exceeds 27 ppm for more than eight hours a day; Denver, 21 ppm; New York City, 16 ppm. Cigarette smoke contains about 400 ppm (one pack per day). This statistic raises the possibility that health symptoms could be related to CO poisoning.

STATISTICS

Each year, according to the Consumer Product Safety Commission, there are more than 200 carbon monoxide deaths related to the use of all types of combustion appliances in the home. The Canadian Medical Association, in a 1979–1988 study, announced that half the fatal poisonings in the United States are attributable to carbon monoxide. Carbon monoxide is the leading cause of death by poisoning in the United States today. Most deaths occur during the winter months, and most occur while victims are sleeping.

Many people have gone to physicians with flu symptoms. In a study compiled by Michael Dolan, M.D. in the *Annals of Emergency Medicine,* 1987, 23.6 percent of those tested with flu symptoms had CO poisoning. Unless a doctor actually tests for CO in the blood, he or she may misdiagnose the illness. This could prove fatal if the CO problem still exists when the patient returns home.

Frequently, carbon monoxide poisoning creates media headlines. The Stevens Point *Wisconsin Journal* of December 19, 1991, reported that an improperly installed ventilation system caused the carbon monoxide leak that emptied a Stevens Point hotel. More than 70 hotel guests and employees were treated at St. Michael's Hospital. Carbon monoxide levels were measured at 450 ppm that night. Anything above 10 ppm is considered dangerous, according to Wisconsin public service workers.

In the winter of 1993–1994, WVIT-TV in Hartford, Connecticut, reported the death of several schoolchildren attending a slumber party. They succumbed to CO poisoning. Backdrafting from the heating system was suspected in this tragedy and in a housing project in Raleigh, North Carolina, where a mother and child were killed. There are no residential performance specifications for flue draft equipment or carbon monoxide levels in the code, although such could be easily written.

A simple repair to a broken vent atop a small furnace could have prevented a family from dying in their one-story home in 1992. The metal rooftop furnace flue vent had come loose and fumes, normally vented out the roof, had poured into the house, causing another CO poisoning.

Gas appliances, unless properly cleaned and maintained, can also pose a hazard. Researchers at the University of California Lawrence Berkeley Laboratory found that cooking with a gas stove at 350° F in a poorly ventilated kitchen could contaminate the room with the same levels of carbon monoxide and nitrogen dioxide gas as is found in the smoggy skies of Los Angeles. Levels of carbon monoxide in homes without gas stoves vary from 0.5 to 5 ppm. Levels near properly adjusted gas stoves are often 5 to 15 ppm, and those near poorly adjusted stoves may be 30 ppm or higher.

Houses that have been weather-tightened for energy efficiency, limiting the entrance of fresh air, can experience backdrafting. This occurs when exhaust fans, clothes dryers and fireplaces create negative pressure which can cause furnace fumes to draw down the flue pipe into the house. Solutions can be as easy as opening a window or, more energy efficient, installing an air-to-air heat exchanger.

Just what is backdrafting? Canadian research into indoor air quality problems revealed an alarming number of backdrafting carbon monoxide poisoning episodes into well-insulated houses with gas, propane or oil-fired heating appliances. Chimneys were partly to blame. Occupants of these energy-efficient houses can suffer from persistent, sometimes bizarre, problems with their chimneys.

Complaints include constant cold downdrafts, combustion gas odors, burnt and melted finishes on heating appliances and even frost buildup on flue pipes in basements. These problems can be attributed to excess house depressurization. This happens when household venting systems such as exhaust fans and fireplaces suck air out of the house, lowering the indoor air pressure relative to the outside. The greater the exhaust capacity and the tighter the building envelope, the more a house is depressurized.

As the house depressurizes, the chimney flow reverses or backdrafts. Outdoor air is sucked down the chimney into the house where it provides air for the exhaust fans, fireplace or whatever. If the exhaust stack for the furnace uses this chimney, gases can spill back into the house for as long as the house is depressurized and the furnace is firing. Hazards from chimney spillage are carbon monoxide, sulfur dioxide and trace elements. Even wood smoke contains unburnt organic matter and vapors. Most are harmless, but some, like benzene, are known to increase the risk of cancer.

Carbon monoxide poisoning has been ranked with syphilis, tuberculosis and subdural hematoma in its ability to mimic a variety of systemic diseases. The most common misdiagnosis of subacute carbon monoxide poisoning is flulike viral illness. The chart below indicates results from a study of patients with elevated COhb (carboxyhemoglobin), above 10 percent.

Age	Race/Sex		Complaint	Diagnosis	COhb
65	B	F	Nausea, cough	Urinary infection	17
32	B	M	General malaise	Viral syndrome	21
61	B	M	Fever, cough	Active TB (lung)	12
42	B	F	Headache	Tension headache	14
56	B	F	Shortness of breath Fever, cough	Bronchitis	15
34	B	F	Headaches, abdominal cramps	Drug-induced headache	11
36	B	M	Weakness, dizziness, cough	Viral syndrome	14
56	W	M	Shortness of breath, cough	Bronchitis	12
71	W	F	Headache, fever	Urinary tract infection Vasovagal headache	11
38	B	F	Headache		11
31	B	M	Abdominal pain	Gastritis	13
33	W	F	Right upper quadrant pain	Biliary colic	10
50	B	F	Weakness, fatigue	Orthostatic hypotension secondary to diuretic use	18

Reprinted from the July, 1987, *Annals of Emergency Medicine.*

DETECTION

If someone in your family has suddenly started having angina symptoms, or if someone seems to be suffering from the "flu" and your doctor has been unable to find the cause, you might want to check the concentration of carbon monoxide in your home. This is especially true if you have a gas-burning appliance inside or even in a garage or room adjacent to your home.

A simple CO disc (approximately $5) placed in your home could easily identify a dangerous problem. There are also permanent CO detectors, similar to smoke alarms, that automatically warn you when CO concentrations are too high.

SOLUTIONS

If you have only mild symptoms of poisoning, get fresh air immediately and eliminate the source of the carbon monoxide. If the symptoms are severe, and your doctor feels it is necessary, you will be treated in a hyperbaric chamber. This unit pushes pure oxygen at high pressure into the body at 20 times the normal rate. However, these units are not readily available and transportation may be needed to reach them. If that is the case, it may be necessary to use an ambulance or air ambulance that is equipped with 100 percent oxygen breathing tanks.

Make sure your home is well-ventilated. Consider installing a heat recovery ventilator if you own a tight house. If you suspect you are being subjected to carbon monoxide poisoning, get fresh air immediately and contact a doctor at once for a proper diagnosis. Choose vented appliances whenever possible.

Watch for a persistent yellow-tipped flame on unvented kerosene or gas space heaters. This is an indicator of maladjustment and increased pollutant emissions. Open a door from the room where space heaters are operating. Install and use exhaust fans vented to the outside over gas cooking stoves and ranges and keep the burners properly adjusted. Make sure the flue is open when using your gas fireplace. Do not vent gas clothes dryers or water heaters into the house. Make sure doors in wood stoves are tight fitting and never use pressure treated or painted wood for fuel as they release chemical pollutants such as arsenic or lead.

Use hardwoods for fireplace burning because they burn hotter and form less creosote, an oily, black tar that sticks to chimneys and stovepipes. Have central air-handling systems, including furnaces, flues and chimneys, inspected annually and promptly repair cracks or damaged parts.

For combustion problems owed to backdrafting, the following precautions should be taken by builders:

1. Label fireplaces with a recommendation to provide additional air during operation
2. Provide a large warm-air register in the furnace room
3. Make sure the chimney is tight by taping the flue connector joints and sealing cracks in the vertical chimney
4. Provide a large dampered air supply duct directly into the lower front floor of the fireplace
5. Tape the cold-air return ducts in the furnace room and also any warm air ducts in crawl spaces or attics
6. Upgrade the thermal performance of furnace and water heater chimneys by using double-walled pipe for the flue connector and an insulated pipe or liner for the vertical chimney
7. Install a heat-recovery ventilation system to balance ventilation
8. Install sealed combustion appliances.

Moffatt, *Progressive Builder*, Dec., 1986.

OTHER POLLUTANTS FROM COMBUSTION DEVICES

Nitrogen dioxide and sulfur dioxide can come from the same burning devices that release carbon monoxide. These pollutants may cause eye, nose, throat and respiratory symptoms, including shortness of breath. Children and individuals with respiratory illnesses such as asthma may be more susceptible to the effects of nitrogen dioxide and sulfur dioxide than adults or those in good health. When asthmatics inhale low levels of these pollutants while exercising, their lung airways can narrow and react more readily to inhaled materials. Evidence from animal studies indicates that exposure to elevated nitrogen dioxide levels may lead, or contribute to, the development of lung diseases such as emphysema.

Respirable particles are released when fuels are incompletely burned; they can lodge in the lungs and irritate or damage lung tissue. The health implications of inhaling particles depend on many factors, including the size of the particles and their chemical makeup. A number of pollutants, including radon and benzo(a)pyrene, both of which can cause cancer, attach to small inhaled particles and are carried deep into the lungs. The risk of lung cancer increases with the amount and length of exposure.

Combustion may also release other pollutants, including unburned hydrocarbons and aldehydes. Little is known about the levels of these pollutants in indoor air or the resulting health effects. Also released in the burning process are formaldehyde, hydrogen cyanide, nitric oxide and vapors from various organic chemicals.

Additional recommendations to reduce noxious fumes follow:
- Buy only combustion appliances that have been tested and certified to meet current safety standards. Change filters in combustion systems on a regular basis. Consider buying appliances that have electronic ignitions rather than pilot lights.
- Never ignore a safety device when it shuts off an appliance. Never ignore the smell of fuel; it usually indicates that an appliance is not operating properly or is leaking fuel. Shut off the appliance, open the windows and call for service. Do not idle the car inside of the garage.

Good News

Organizations such as the Underwriters Laboratories and the American Gas Association Laboratories certify combustion appliances that have been tested and that meet current safety standards. These appliances are labeled for consumers.

The U.S. Consumer Product Safety Commission selected carbon monoxide, fuel gas detection and smoke detection as priority projects for fiscal year 1992. The aims of these projects, including the promotion of the development of reliable, low-cost CO and fuel gas detectors and smoke alarms for consumer use, appear to have been realized as these types of units have recently appeared on the market.

Industry standards require all currently manufactured vented gas heaters to have a safety shutoff device. This device helps protect from carbon monoxide poisoning by shutting off an improperly vented heater.

Heaters made after 1982 have a pilot light safety system called an oxygen depletion sensor. This system shuts off a heater when there is not enough fresh air, before the heater begins producing large amounts of carbon monoxide. Look for the label that tells you that the appliance has this safety system. Electronic ignitions are more efficient and eliminate the continuous low-level pollutants from pilot lights. All new wood stoves are EPA-certified to limit the amounts of pollutants released into the outdoor air.

In 1988 the Consumer Product Safety Commission recalled the Preway Arkla high-efficiency furnace because of corrosion problems in the heat exchanger which allowed fumes to leak into homes. As a result, the newest generation of furnaces has improved safety devices to prevent catastrophe by using stainless steel in secondary heat exchangers and high-performance plastics in the venting system.

Combustion Appliances and Potential Problems

Appliances	Fuel	Potential Problem
Central furnaces	Gas	Cracked heat exchanger
	Oil	Cracked heat exchanger
Coal stoves	Coal	Same as oil/gas, including defective grate
Room heaters	Gas	Inadequate air for burning
	Wood	Inadequate air for burning and green or treated wood
	Kerosene	Improper adjustment, wrong fuel (not K-1), wrong wick or wick height
Fireplaces	Gas	Defective/blocked flue, maladjusted burner
	Coal	Defective/blocked flue, green or treated wood, cracked heat exchanger or firebox

Appliances	Fuel	Potential Problem
Central heaters	Wood	Inadequate air for burning, green or treated wood
	Kerosene	Improper adjustment, wrong fuel (not K-1), wrong wick or wick height, improper air for burning
Water heaters	Gas	Improper air for burning, defective/blocked flue, mal-adjusted burner
Ranges	Gas	Improper air for burning, maladjusted burner, misuse as room heater
Stoves	Wood	Improper air for burning

Combustion Appliances and Indoor Air Pollution, Consumer Product Safety Commission.

FOR MORE INFORMATION

American Gas Association, 1515 Wilson Boulevard, Arlington, Virginia 22209

Canadian Mortgage and Housing Corporation Study, CMHC, 682 Montreal Road, Ottawa, Ontario, Canada K1A 0P7

Carbon Monoxide Safety & Health Association 1-800-432-5599, 11211 Sorrento Valley Road, Suite D, San Diego, California 92121

Gas Appliance Manufacturers Association, 1901 N. Moore Street, Arlington, Virginia 22209

National Kerosene Heater Association (615) 269-9015

Straight Answers to Burning Questions, Wood Burning Alliance, 1101 Connecticut Avenue NW, Suite 700, Washington, DC 20036

"What You Should Know About Space Heaters," "What You Should Know About Kerosene Heaters," U.S. Consumer Product Safety Commission, Washington, DC 20207

Wood Heater Program, EPA, 401 M Street SW, Washington, DC 20460

ELECTRO-MAGNETIC STRESS

IN RECENT TIMES there has been much controversy about the effect of electromagnetic flux on the human condition. It is difficult to measure the effect as there are so many factors to consider.

Looking into nature, one can observe other creatures involved with the electrical process. There are many living organisms that actually create electrical phenomena. For example, the electric eel has the power to generate substantial amounts of direct current through an electrochemical process, as compared with our electromechanical systems. Then there is the firefly who generates electroluminescent light. Each creature generates electrical phenomena for its own purpose: either defense, mating or hunting.

We generate electrical phenomena for many purposes. But it was not long ago that we did none of this. Electricity is a "Johnny-come-lately" for the human race. Now we have the use of it, however, through the work of Franklin, Edison, Tesla, Faraday, Curie and so many others.

We have always been surrounded by magnetic fields and other radiation. Now we have added to natural conditions with our unnatural ones through the use of radio, television, radar, cellular phones, generating plants, microwaves, computers, home wiring and even electric blankets.

Why should we be concerned? We are also made with electrical operating systems that are basically electrochemical in nature. The entire procedure of moving a finger involves an electrochemical reaction in the brain in which a group of neurons discharge electrical energy to create an electrical communications path along a line of nerve systems which end up activating a muscle. All this is contingent on the proper functioning of a carbon-based wiring system in the human body. It is also based on noninterference from the outside.

This is where the multitude of rampant electrical signals comes in. We were never as deluged with the spectrum of electrical impulses and forces as we are today. Our newfound technology has the feature of spilling signals and power into our private body areas without our permission, and without our knowledge. By the time that we have caught up with the symptoms, we are already in severe danger. The message is that we must continue to be alert, to maintain research and act appropriately and in a timely manner.

DESCRIPTION

An extremely low frequency (ELF) electromagnetic field is not radiation, but captive electric and magnetic fields that are generated by strong electric current in power appliances. The two types of fields, electric and magnetic, are related. Electric fields generate voltage and are easy to shield by using conductive materials. Magnetic fields generate a current (amperage) measured in a unit called a "gauss" and are difficult to shield against.

Electromagnetic stress is metabolic disruption caused by electromagnetic interference. Our bodies produce millions of electrical impulses within our highly developed bioelectrochemical magnetic fields. These balance and regulate the activity of our cells. Our bodies are constantly interacting with man-made random electromagnetic fields (EMF's) generated by electrical wiring, electronics, appliances, computers and telecommunication networks, in addition to microwave and power transmission lines. These random signals interpenetrate body tissues and alter the electromagnetic functions. The resultant disruption causes a host of symptoms which are normally diagnosed as being caused by other factors.

An average alternating (AC) current inside the body of about one-billionth of an amp per square centimeter seems to be the conservative threshold for biological effects. Very preliminary results show that at five times that level, an increase in protein production in cancer cells is seen; but when the field is increased a thousand times further, the increase in protein production is only three times greater. These results suggest that it is better to spend a short time well above the 60Hz threshold (3 milligauss) than a long time just above it. (A milligauss is a unit of measurement for electromagnetic fields recorded on appropriate instruments called gaussmeters.)

In laboratory studies, conclusions were reached that showed heart rates slowed with exposure to moderate levels of electromagnetic fields, but not with high or low levels. This would indicate that there may be a "window" of exposure that is more harmful than strictly high doses, but abnormal, man-made electromagnetic fields, regardless of their frequencies, produce the same biological effects.

They have had demonstrated effects on the calcium channel permeability of cell membranes, which can affect a variety of cell functions including the transmission of electric signals to the nerve tissue. These effects, which deviate from normal functions and may be harmful, are the following:

- Increase in the rate of cancer-cell division
- Increase in the incidence of certain cancers
- Developmental abnormalities in embryos
- Alterations in neurochemicals resulting in behavioral abnormalities such as suicide
- Alterations in biological cycles
- Stress responses in exposed animals that, if prolonged, lead to declines in immune-system efficiency
- Alterations in learning ability

R.O. Becker, *Cross Currents*, 1990.

Microwave Health Risks
Greater than 5mW/2

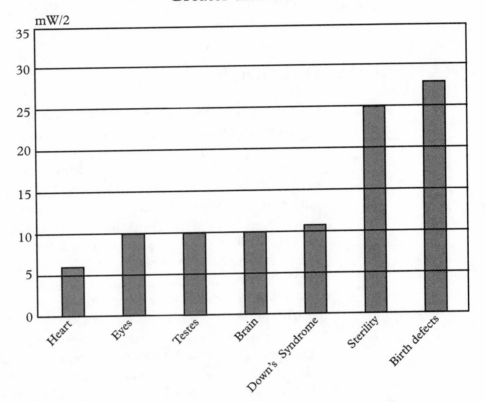

Bodily functions most affected are those which are most active at night: electrical meridians that regulate the liver, gallbladder, lungs and large intestine. During sleep, the normal detoxification process is blocked by electromagnetic (EM) stress on those meridians. In order to reduce EM effects it is necessary to consider eliminating current from appliances in the bedroom, including electric blankets, waterbed heaters and clock radios.

Magnetic fields which affect body tissue are not blocked by common building materials or walls, and exist on both the inside and outside of your home. One thing to keep in mind is that electromagnetic radiation goes through wood and other usual building materials. If a TV set is placed with its back against an inside wall, radiation will be present in the adjoining room, just as if there were no wall present. Consequently, an infant or child's bed should not be placed against a wall adjacent to a TV set, regardless of the set's field strength. A safe distance must be kept from EM-radiating appliances in a 360° circle, not just from the front of the unit.

STATISTICS AND STUDIES

In addition to the hazards of radiation leakage from defective microwave ovens, EMF's in the microwave range (length of wave frequency) are being studied. As disclosed in *Cross Currents* by R.O. Becker, Dr. Sam Koslov, director of the Applied Physics Laboratory at Johns Hopkins University, presented preliminary results of a microwave-exposure study. At an EPA-sponsored public meeting on environmental electromagnetic fields, Koslov reported a possible link between Alzheimer's disease and microwave exposure. Koslov, who has been associated with the electromagnetic bioeffects field since the 1940's, studied the effects of microwave exposure on the eyes of chimpanzees.

The animals were exposed repeatedly to low-level, nonthermal microwaves, and their eyes were regularly examined. As the study progressed, one animal began to demonstrate the classic clinical signs of Alzheimer's disease. On autopsy, the animal's brain showed the typical pathological picture associated with Alzheimer's disease. Koslov stated that he was revealing this information to the public out of frustration with the lack of funding for the area of electromagnetic bioeffects. Microwaves can cook living creatures from the inside out and have been implicated as a cause of cataracts, as these beams can penetrate moderate distances through living tissue.

Overhead power lines have been a source of epidemiological study for many years. In 1992 an electromagnetic field research study of half a million people in Sweden at the Karolinska Institute of Environmental Medicine in Stockholm concluded that living near power lines increased the leukemia rate in children by about four times over normal incidence. In adults, cancers were one and a half to three times more likely to occur.

Researchers found a twofold increase in childhood leukemias associated with powerline fields of 1-2 milligauss, a threefold increase with 3 milligauss fields, and a fourfold increase with higher fields. Also, a study of 252 Denver, Colorado, leukemia cases linked power lines to childhood cancers.

In the United States, a Boston University researcher claims that people who say they live near transmission lines are twice as likely to show symptoms of depression as those who do not.

The Syracuse, New York, Veterans Administration Hospital reports that plant growth is stunted as far away as 1,000 feet from power lines. Also at that distance, behavioral effects, like decreases in human reaction time, are observed, and people living closer than that distance had changes in their blood chemistry and electrocardiograms.

Computer technology has also been studied for harmful EMF effects. In the *American Journal of Epidemiology*, November 1, 1992, a study showed that women working at computer terminals that exposed them to more than three milligauss of ELF's (the minimum safe level is considered to be three milligauss or less) had three and a half times the risk of miscarriage as women who worked at low-emitting visual display terminals (VDT's). *The International Journal of Cancer*, May, 1992, published a study that found an almost fivefold increase in brain tumors among women who worked at VDT's.

In the *American Journal of Industrial Medicine*, June, 1988, a study found a double rate of miscarriage among women who used VDT's more than 20 hours per week. The biggest problem with all these studies is the number of variables that could have altered the results, such as stress, home ELF environment, diet, etc. However, laboratory studies have shown a definite ELF effect on test subjects which could contribute to increased miscarriages, even if they were not the sole cause.

After a study by the U.S. National Institute for Occupational Safety and Health (NIOSH) (*New England Journal of Medicine*, March 14, 1991) reported no increased miscarriage risk among telephone operators who use VDT's, articles appeared in the popular press saying the pregnancy risk had been disproved. However, the NIOSH study has been widely criticized because it compared VDT users with a control group of women—telephone operators who used a different type of equipment—who were exposed to the same levels of ELF magnetic fields as the test group.

Studies in the United States found significantly increased cancer rates associated with exposure to power line fields in the

2.5 milligauss range. Beginning in 1986, researchers began to investigate the field effects of both high- and low-frequency electromagnetic radiation on human health and physiology. This group found that eyestrain, stress and fatigue were associated with VDT emission.

In July, 1991, the Swedish government implemented a new standard requiring that ELF magnetic emissions from computer monitors not exceed 2.5 milligauss at 19.7 inches from the screen. The Swedish labor union did their own investigation and determined that the standard should be 2.0 milligauss at 11.8 inches. This standard has been adopted by the New York City Board of Education, which requires that all new monitors purchased by the New York City school system conform to these standards. Most manufacturers are now selling low EMF computer screens. A list of these models and their manufacturers is given below, showing the maximum VLF (very low frequency) emissions for each.

Computer monitors	Max. VLF emissions (in nanoteslas)
ACS ACM-1540-UT	17.00
Addonics C152/LR	17.40
ADI MicroScan 3GP	18.20
ADI MicroScan 4GP	17.40
CTX 1581LR	13.20
Darius HRN-14VLP	12.20
Darius HRN-15VLP	15.00
Digital PCXBV-BC	12.60
Digital PCXBV-DE	15.20
ETCViewMagic CA-1464SP	8.20
ETCViewMagic CA-1565SP	14.00
GoldStar Model 1510	13.80
IBM 14P Color	12.60
IBM 15P Color	14.60
KFC CA-1508	15.00
KFC CM-1428MD2	12.00
Liberty CL-9015	10.60
Mitsubishi Diamond Scan 15FS	14.80
Nanao FlexScan F240iW	12.60
NEC MultiSync 3V	18.20
NEC MultiSync 4FGe	11.60
Nokia Multigraph 448S	17.40

Computer monitors	Max. VLF emissions *(in nanoteslas)*
Nokia Multigraph 449E	9.40
Optiquest 1500D	17.20
Packard Bell PB8549SVGL	16.80
Philips Brilliance 15	14.80
Sampo AlphaScan 15e	15.20
Samtron SC528UXL	11.80
Sceptre CC-615L	13.60
Sony CPD-1430	16.80
ViewSonic 15	14.60
ZDS ZCM-1440-UT	8.80

Hazardous health effects from EMF's can be varied and can come from many sources.

An Oregon physician was in the habit of wearing a beeper on his left side. Neither he nor his personal physician realized the potential significance of this source of electromagnetic fields so close to the body. The doctor developed a chronic inflammation in his left foot. Neither natural nor allopathic treatments would get rid of it. Only when the author identified the connection between the beeper location and its electromagnetic stress field on precisely the same acupuncture meridian as the inflamed area of the foot was improvement possible. The acupuncture meridians carry not only a flow of energy, but also metabolic waste products. The flow is driven by the body's own electromagnetic field. When a much stronger field is superimposed, it can block the flow of the meridian, resulting in energy imbalances, functional disturbances and toxicity buildup. Over longer periods of time, clinical disease is the result.*

Common electric appliances are culprits as well. Using an electric razor regularly may boost a man's risk of developing leukemia because the razors are used on the facial skin near to the pineal gland in the brain. It is speculated that the magnetic field might suppress the pineal gland's production of a hormone believed to help the body protect itself against cancer. Hair dry-

*G. Swarthout, *Electromagnetic Pollution Solutions*, AERI Publishing, 1991.

Milligauss Levels
In contact with the object

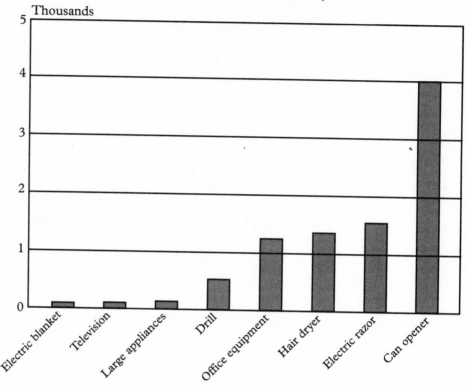

ers also put out extreme levels of EMF's, which may not harm the occasional user, but are definitely hazardous to the professional beautician who uses them constantly.

Television sets and corresponding video games should have warning labels affixed to them. Viewers should maintain a safe distance of at least three feet from the standard size set and more than three feet from larger screens. This does not apply to projection television screens as they do not contain cathode-ray tubes. Clock radios, fax machines, copiers and phone answering machines should all be kept a safe distance from the user.

Since most of us spend six to eight hours in one place during sleep, it is important not to have any health hazards that affect us repeatedly. EMF's from wiring, electric blankets, waterbed heaters, fans, etc. can be dangerous, as these fields impinge on the pineal gland, suppressing production of the hormone melatonin, produced by the gland. This can cause the liver to be unable to achieve its proper nighttime detoxification mode. Blankets and heaters must be unplugged at night to avoid any residual current. Use them only to warm the bed, unless you feel safe with one of the new low-EMF blankets.

In an interview with Cyril Smith, Ph.D., in the October, 1992, issue of *Mastering Food Allergies*, the effect of ambient EMF's on human health was discussed. It was noted that the endocrine system is regulated by hormones and other biochemical factors from the cerebral cortex, the hypothalamus, the hippocampus and the pineal gland, and that these brain areas are all highly sensitive and electrically active. A pulsing low-intensity EMF (one that is cycling on and off) will cause a release of noradrenaline in most people within 15 minutes; this may result in an increase in hospital admissions during times of magnetic disturbance. According to Dr. Smith, many people not sick enough to be hospitalized would still not feel well in a variety of nonspecific ways.

Television and microwave towers also have been targets of studies. The Federal Communications Commission (FCC) emissions figures from TV towers show that the radiation level within a one-mile radius of a major TV broadcasting tower can be ten times higher than the limit the former Soviet Union considered safe for its citizens. In Florida, residents are fighting cable companies who want to make a deal with public schools to install their towers in school backyards. The residents claim this could give their children long-term health problems. The companies say the towers are safe, and the debate continues.

DETECTION

Measurement devices include electrostress meters, gauss meters, Tri-field meters and several other indicators readily available from catalogues and eco-stores.

SOLUTION

Obviously, the best answer to EMF's is to remove the field source by turning off appliances, but this is not always possible as we live in a powered world. There is one place where you can ensure an EMF-free environment . . . your bedroom at night. Install a bedroom cutoff demand switch which removes power to wiring while you sleep. If you need an electric clock alarm, leave that plug on a separate circuit and place it as far from your sleeping place as possible.

When considering new construction, look into shielded wiring as an answer to containing EMF fields in your home. Also, do not design the placement of a bedroom or work space near any electric service panels or junction boxes.

If you must use a computer, investigate new products that reduce harmful EMF emissions. Install a device to reduce magnetic fields transmitted from computer monitors, the most effective being a cathode-ray tube shield. If unable to do this, install a long cord to a portable keyboard and sit three to four feet away from the monitor. This may make it difficult to read the screen, but using a magnifier attachment will solve the problem. The best solution is to purchase one of the new monitors with low EMF emissions.

Remember, EMF emissions are 360 degrees and normally stronger at the back of the unit than the front. This means that you must maintain a good distance (measuring with a gaussmeter or the like) from the wall or divider where another computer may be in operation.

Other office equipment producing high EMF are copiers, fax machines and phone answering machines. Cellular phones and beepers can also affect their users, depending on the type and construction of the units. Before purchasing any unit, contact the manufacturer and ask for a report on the EMF output.

To safeguard your children, do not allow them to spend excessive time using electronic toys and instruct them to sit three to four feet back from television sets, including when they are using video games. If they play computer games, school them in proper computer distance or install appropriate protection devices.

Protection from electric panels and structurally embedded EMF sources is currently being developed. Magnetic fields pass virtually unaffected through concrete, water, earth, almost all building materials and most metals (lead aprons will not shield against magnetic fields). Effective shielding requires special ferrous alloys engineered for the purpose, such as mu-metals, iron, nickel and cobalt with special heat treatment. These can be used to reduce fields to 10 milligauss throughout an office if applied correctly.

Also available is a nonhazardous, low odor, electric field conductive water base paint designed for interior use on wood, plaster and drywall. It is used where effective shielding of electric fields is required. This paint must be grounded as it conducts electricity. It is available from Electro Pollution Supply, (602) 445-8225.

Good News

Some EMF's are being successfully used in the medical profession. Andrew Bassett, an orthopedic surgeon and retired Columbia University medical school professor, predicts that the use of EMF's to treat patients is going to vastly increase in the 1990's. He foresees diabetics being treated with an electric charge instead of insulin. When chemotherapy for head and neck cancers was administered with pulsed EMF's, the therapy was more effective than with conventional administration because the drug became 650,000 times more concentrated in cells. In addition, ELF fields are being used in treating bone fractures. The fields apparently promote bone growth and hasten healing.

Manufacturing is capitalizing on EMF by putting out new products. Newer electric blankets have cut EMF's by 95 percent (Casco's Soft Heat and Northern Electric's Sunbeam and Slumber Rest brands, made after 1990, are low-field products). Field shields for blow dryers, razors and can openers, all sources of high EMF's, are being devised. One manufacturer claims to have created a device that can neutralize the negative effects of electromagnetic radiation fields. Clarus Environmental Systems provides these devices not only for VDT's, but also to clear up chaotic fields in home or office.

In late 1992 Congress passed a far-reaching national energy bill that, among many other provisions, authorizes an electromagnetic field research and public information program. The EPA is considering resuming work on setting safety limits for human exposures to radio frequency and microwave (RF/MW) radiation. They had discontinued this work in 1988.

The U.S. Congress has directed the National Institute for Occupational Safety and Health to begin an epidemiological study of the possible link between police radar use and cancer.

Big business also is recognizing the hazards of EMF's in the workplace. Several major corporations recently identified floor-level magnetic fields of 150 to 300 milligauss generated by power cables or electrical switching gear. They employed shielding methods at great expense to alleviate the problem and protect their employees.

FORMALDEHYDE

SONIA HALL IS a formaldehyde casualty. She sued the manufacturer of the particleboard that caused her trauma and won. The formaldehyde hazard can cause physical effects that last a lifetime.

In March of 1989, Sonia and her husband Terry decided to have their carpets cleaned in their home, which was only ten years old. They returned home after the cleaning service had completed their job, and within two hours Sonia began to have an uneasy feeling. Her symptoms became more intense and seemed to vary depending on the humidity level. Since there was a noticeable smell remaining, the Halls called in the cleaners to rinse the carpets again.

The smell only got worse, as did Sonia's symptoms, which included mental disorientation, confusion, shortness of breath, fatigue, tight throat and burning in the digestive tract.

She could only get relief by sleeping in the bathroom. Her doctor treated her for a multitude of disorders and her friends chided her as a hypochondriac. Her condition cleared up when she spent extended periods of time away from her home and resurfaced when she returned. By process of elimination, the Halls determined that the problem was coming from the flooring. Terry pulled up the carpet and found that the underlay was particleboard and the subfloor, plywood. He immediately hired a laboratory to perform an air test; it confirmed a 4 to 10 parts per million level of formaldehyde in the home (recommended levels are .01 ppm).

Terry replaced the subfloor with exterior grade plywood

which uses a different type of formaldehyde glue and sealed it with a nontoxic sealant. Hardwood flooring was installed and the home was retested, with the results at acceptable levels. Sonia could now live in the house, but she still exhibited symptoms, especially when she went to public places. She was diagnosed as having organic brain syndrome and sought help from her allergist. Shortly after the testing she went into anaphylactic shock and almost died. The tests proved she was now allergic to a whole list of airborne contaminants. Sonia entered into a program to desensitize her. Many doctors later, she found Dr. Alan Lieberman in Charleston, South Carolina. He has effectively reduced her symptoms with a variety of methods including "sauna treatment."

Sonia still must be careful where she goes. During her court hearing against the manufacturer she became so ill from the air in the courtroom that she collapsed. The manufacturer stated that there was a defect in the glue process that held the particleboard together. This allowed water from the cleaning process to partially dissolve the glue and allowed formaldehyde fumes to outgas. A company chemist stated that this glue was known to affect people with certain allergies, asthma or chemical sensitivities, but that there was no requirement to place labeling on the product or notify the builders using the product.

Sonia still tests positive for high levels of formaldehyde in her blood and still exhibits symptoms from time to time, although treatment has reduced the severity of these. Modern medicine claims she cannot be cured. Some of the symptoms she encountered were heart pain, hypertension, edema, chest and lung fullness, asthma, fatigue, post trauma stress, mental confusion, stiffness of shoulders, arms and hips and bronchitis.

DESCRIPTION

Formaldehyde is a colorless, gaseous chemical compound that is generally present at low, variable concentrations in both indoor and outdoor air. Formaldehyde by itself, or in combination with other chemicals, serves a number of purposes in manufactured products. It is emitted by many construction materials and consumer products that contain formaldehyde-based glues, resins, preservatives and bonding agents. Formaldehyde also is an ingredient in home insulation foam used until the early 1980's.

Formaldehyde can be found in a multitude of products including glue, adhesive, paint preservatives and pressed wood products made with urea-formaldehyde resins such as particleboard and hardwood plywood paneling, medium density fiberboard (for drawer fronts and cabinets), exterior strand board and UFFI (urea-formaldehyde foam insulation). Sources of formaldehyde in the home include smoke, household products and unvented fuel-burning appliances such as gas stoves or kerosene space heaters.

Many textile products are treated with formaldehyde. Permanent press finishes are added to clothing and draperies. Even when not stated on the label, all polyester/cotton-blend fabrics have formaldehyde finishes. Polyester/cotton bed sheets have a particularly heavy finish because of their continuous use and frequent laundering. Formaldehyde is also used on nylon fabrics to make them flameproof. Some pure-cotton fabrics have also been treated with formaldehyde finishes for easy care.

Even though it is not required by law that a manufacturer indicate the finish chemical or the care characteristics, clothing labels may state that a finish is "permanent pressed," "no-iron," "crease resistant," "shrink proof," "stretch proof," "water repellent," "waterproof," or "permanently pleated." These finishes combine formaldehyde resin directly with the fiber, making the formaldehyde "permanent." Washing can lower the formaldehyde levels, but formaldehyde continues to be released as the resin breaks down during washing, ironing and wear.

Formaldehyde in most substances is most toxic when the materials are new, as emissions decrease with age (particularly over the first two or three years). Therefore, it is difficult to identify this culprit unless you perform a formaldehyde test.

Your health can be affected in many ways by this toxic component. It can cause watery eyes, burning sensations in the eyes and throat, nausea, skin rash, cough, tiredness, excessive thirst, nosebleeds, insomnia, disorientation and difficulty in breathing (at levels above 0.1 ppm). High concentrations may trigger attacks in asthmatics. Formaldehyde has been shown to cause cancer in animals and may also cause cancer in humans. If ingested, it can cause nausea, vomiting, clammy skin and other symptoms of shock, severe abdominal pain, internal bleeding, loss of ability to urinate, vertigo and coma. A preliminary study speculates that formaldehyde may be a contributing factor in sudden infant death syndrome.

STATISTICS AND STUDIES

It is estimated that 10 to 20 percent of the general population may be susceptible to the irritant properties of formaldehyde, even at extremely low concentrations.

Most wood products today are made of particleboard or plywood instead of solid wood. Particleboard, made from small wood shavings with formaldehyde resin and pressed into a woodlike form, is easily recognizable because the pressed-together shavings can be seen on all sides. Plywood's cross section shows several sheets of wood sandwiched together with phenol-formaldehyde resin.

Particleboard warning labels state, "This product is manufactured with a urea-formaldehyde resin and will release small quantities of formaldehyde. Formaldehyde levels in the indoor air can cause temporary eye and respiratory irritation and may aggravate respiratory conditions or allergies. Ventilation will reduce indoor formaldehyde levels."

Use of formaldehyde compounds is widespread in the manufacture of furniture, cabinets, and other building materials. When products are new, high indoor temperatures or humidity can cause increased release of formaldehyde from these products.

Outgassing is most severe when a product is new, so it is a good idea to ventilate buildings well during construction. Phenol formaldehyde (PF) resins are synthesized from petroleum (phenol) and natural gas (formaldehyde).

These additives may be tolerable on the outside of your walls. None outgas as much as the urea-formaldehyde resins used in most interior paneling products.

Standard interior wallboard (drywall, sheetrock) has also reportedly irritated some ultrasensitive patients. Whether the trouble arises from the plaster, the glue that binds the surface paper or the joint compound is undetermined.

Reports of health problems stemming from formaldehyde exposure are not uncommon. In a 1978 article, the *Medical Tribune* reported that Russian studies showed that factory workers exposed daily to formaldehyde at a concentration of 1.6 ppm became irritable and unable to sleep. Yet, one family in Connecticut was found to be living in a home atmosphere of 27 ppm. In 1978 a writer for the *Hartford Courant* uncovered more than 20 families suffering from formaldehyde-induced illness in Connecticut alone.

In 1978 Peter A. Breysse, a University of Washington assistant professor in environmental health who had been studying the problem, reported that many mobile home owners had been undergoing treatment for "mysterious ailments" for years with little success; at the time, neither patients nor doctors were aware of formaldehyde exposure. In New York, a doctor was reportedly unable to work in his office for several weeks after urea-formaldehyde was foamed into his walls. Whenever he tried, his eyes, throat and nose became irritated and his head began to ache.

A *Popular Science* reader sent a letter to the editor after reading an article on the composition of new wood materials. He had used composition boards made from wood by-products laminated with phenolic resins when he renovated his basement. He discovered that about 5 to 20 percent of his visitors to the completed recreation room developed allergic reactions ranging from mild to severe eye tearing or burning. Only a complete periodic ventilation alleviated the problem. Covering or otherwise sealing some of the particleboard helped as well.

DETECTION

If you are considering new construction, contact the builder to see if the materials contain formaldehyde. If the builder does not know, contact the manufacturer.

In an existing structure, identify the presence of the toxin through a self-test kit available from catalogues and eco-stores, or contact a local lab and have them inspect your home with proper testing equipment.

Homes with no new materials or furnishings added after three years may not have toxic levels of formaldehyde as the emissions decrease with time, but think twice when buying furnishings or decorating materials. Also, avoid buying clothes or furnishings labeled wash and wear unless you can verify that they do not contain formaldehyde.

SOLUTIONS

Obviously, if you do not purchase formaldehyde-based products, you won't be susceptible to their toxic effects. If your home tests positive for formaldehyde and you cannot remove the material, consider purchasing an air filtration device that absorbs this substance (activated carbon). Also consider installing a heat recovery ventilator to provide constant air circulation. Growing spider plants indoors is an easy way to reduce toxic levels as they are absorbers of formaldehyde.

Nontoxic sealers such as Hard Seal, manufactured by AFM, prevent off-gassing from painted and varnished surfaces of materials and dry to a clear finish.

Synthetic carpets can contain formaldehyde. If they are already installed and are less than five years old, treat them with a carpet sealer such as Carpet Guard from AFM. If you are in the market for a new rug, consider wool, cotton or one of the new synthetics made without harsh chemicals or adhesives.

The rate at which formaldehyde is released is accelerated by heat and may also depend somewhat on the humidity level. Therefore, the use of dehumidifiers and air-conditioning to control humidity and to maintain a moderate temperature can help reduce formaldehyde emissions.

Buy cabinets made of real wood or metal, which may be difficult to find. A good substitute is a wood-faced cabinet with particleboard shelves and sides that can be covered with a nontoxic sealant. You could also choose exterior grade plywood (instead of interior grade) for countertops and other construction. Exterior grade plywood has less formaldehyde.

For construction, call Medite Corporation (503)779-9596 or Boise Cascade (503)224-7250 to find out where to purchase their formaldehyde-free particleboard. As a safety measure be sure to seal in these products' glues with nontoxic sealants.

Good News

Since 1985 the federal government, through the U.S. Department of Housing and Urban Development, has enforced regulations that sharply curtail the use of materials containing formaldehyde in prefabricated and manufactured homes, limiting use to the lower emitting products.

UFFI is no longer used. Manufacturers are developing products that substitute other compounds for resins and avoid the use of formaldehyde. OSB products that claim to be "formaldehyde free," such as Louisiana Pacific's Inner Seal products, use an isocyanate resin known in the industry as MDI. MDI is wholly derived from natural gas and can be highly toxic until it is cured. After curing, the company considers it stable and safe, although sealing the surfaces or using it for external application would be prudent.

FOR MORE INFORMATION

- "Air Pollution in Your Home," home indoor air quality checklist, from local chapters of the American Lung Association.
- "Formaldehyde: Everything You Wanted to Know but Were Afraid to Ask," Consumer Federation of America, 1424 16th Street NW, Washington, DC 20036 (send addressed, stamped envelope)
- EPA Toxic Substance Control Act assistance line (202) 554-1404

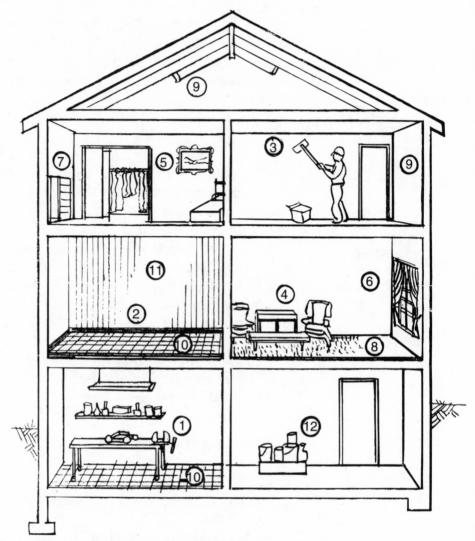

WHERE FORMALDEHYDE MAY BE FOUND IN THE HOME

1. In hobby and workshop areas: glue.
2. Adhesives used to secure flooring.
3. Paint with formaldehyde.
4. Particle board used in some furniture.
5. Wash-and-wear clothing.
6. Stain resistant drapes and furniture upholstery.
7. Cabinets using particle board.
8. Carpets made of artificial materials.
9. UFFI insulation (before 1980).
10. Particle board/plywood underlayment.
11. Particle board photofinish or plywood panelling.
12. Stored paint cans.

LEAD

DESCRIPTION

ONCE EXTRACTED FROM its naturally occurring state as an ore, lead has thousands of applications. Lead's durability, malleability, mass, low melting point and resistance to corrosion from many chemicals make it indispensable for many industries. Lead has no known functions or health benefits for humans and therefore should be regarded as a poison. The following true story illustrates the importance of paying attention to lead in the home.

Wendy and Gordon Brown lived in a new house when their son Nicholas was born. As the family grew, they moved into a 200-year-old house owned by another family member and subsequently into their own 200-year-old country house. They were careful to make sure no toxic materials were used in any decorating they did because they were concerned for the welfare of their children.

Cameron, their second son, was a very shy child, spending numerous hours just sitting, staring off into space and looking at the wall. They noticed he had a coordination problem and did not like to interact with other children very much. Their third child, Jennifer, was born with some problems with brain function and by 15 months she had also developed asthma.

In April of 1993, Wendy viewed a television program about a child who had lead poisoning from paint. She immediately became concerned and called the previous owner of the home to see if there was lead paint in it. The former owner claimed there was no such thing. Not satisfied, Wendy took her daughter to the doctor and had her tested for lead. The results came back at 16 micrograms per deciliter; since the "safe" level is considered 9 or less, the doctor recommended that she be put on a high-iron supplement to reduce the risk of further lead ingestion.

Wendy was determined to find out if her house was responsible for the lead contamination and went to the hardware store to find a lead test. She selected the Lead Zone detector test because it was the most reasonably priced. Upon returning home, she tested all the walls, woodwork, floors and ceilings. To her horror, she found lead paint on all the woodwork and parts of the floor. She had heard that professional remediation costs a small fortune in an older home, and didn't know what to do, so she called the Lead Zone manufacturer, Enzone, and just happened to get the president, Joe MacDonald, on the phone. Joe calmed her down and instructed her to wash the woodwork every other day with trisodium phosphate to keep the dust down. She also was told to damp mop the house and not to vacuum, which was easy because she did not have any carpets. Wendy was concerned with lead in the water, but Gordon figured the old pipes had been replaced with copper. They tested their water anyway, which came back negative. Luckily the walls did not test positive for lead and Wendy even checked them where the plaster had deteriorated.

The Browns could not afford to replace all the woodwork and floors, therefore Joe suggested that they use his paint, Encapsulant, to cover the woodwork. Wendy found it to be a sticky substance that adhered like rubber, but when dry it was an effective way to eliminate further dusting and chipping of lead paint. She still continues to damp mop just in case.

Cameron and Nicholas had also been tested for lead and they came back at 15 and 16 micrograms per deciliter. They also were put on a high-iron program. In seven months Cameron responded well; he became more attentive and started playing with his peers. Nicholas never showed any visible signs of lead poisoning. All children will undergo subsequent testing; if their lead levels go down, Wendy and Gordon will know they have been successful. If the results are not encouraging, they may elect to have their walls x-rayed to see whether lead lurks beneath the surface paint.

The Browns also are planning to investigate the school that Nicholas is attending to see whether any lead-in-water tests have been done and whether the soil in the playground could harbor lead dust. They are concerned that they may cure the problem at home only to have their children poisoned inadvertently throughout their school years.

Wendy and Gordon were lucky that they caught this problem before their children's lead levels increased. They were unaware that Cameron's behavioral abnormalities indicated a possible lead contamination. Their doctor was the first to identify the possibility. Wendy was a conscientious homemaker, but it was the media's report on TV that made her aware enough to take matters into her own hands.

Lead can be found in many places: the air, drinking water, food, contaminated soil, dust, dinnerware, pottery and toys. Also, lead solder found in food containers, faucets and water pipes can leach lead.

Scientists and physicians have reported deleterious health effects stemming from lead, such as damage to the kidneys, liver and nervous system; reproductive, cardiovascular, immune and gastrointestinal systems; and the manufacture of heme (the oxygen-carrying part of hemoglobin in red blood cells), a cause of encephalopathy and degenerative brain disease. Lead is considered to be a metabolic poison that inhibits some of the basic enzymatic functions. Once lead enters the body, it is treated like calcium because the body cannot tell the difference between the two. After several weeks, lead leaves the bloodstream and is absorbed by bone, where it can continue to accumulate over a lifetime.

Children process lead differently than adults, so they absorb up to 50 percent of the lead they ingest. Adults absorb 10 percent. Those under age seven are at greatest risk because their still-developing brains and nervous systems are exquisitely sensitive to even minute amounts of lead. Infants under age one may be most vulnerable of all. Fetuses whose mothers are exposed to high lead levels also can suffer irreversible damage. Lead is extremely toxic, so even 15 parts per billion (about the equivalent of 15 raindrops in an Olympic-size swimming pool) can be dangerous, particularly if consumed regularly by infants in milk or formula.

In children, symptoms of lead toxicity include insomnia, irritability, colic, anemia, damage to intellectual development, arrested growth, decreased hearing acuity and decreased ability to maintain a steady posture. Lead poisoning in children can mean a lower IQ and impairment in reading, writing, math, visual and motor skills, language, abstract thinking and concentration. Severe lead exposure can cause coma, convulsions and even death.

Exposure to lead paint dust is the number one nationwide cause of lead poisoning in children. The danger is greatest in the estimated 57 million American homes painted before 1978, when lead was banned from household paint.

As many as 20 percent of American homes may have elevated lead levels in water. Lead can leach into tap water from lead pipes, connectors or service lines and bronze or brass faucets which contain lead. Even copper pipes can have lead solder. The insides of most faucets are made of bronze or brass (an alloy of copper, zinc and other metallic chemicals), both of which contain lead.

Fresh fruit and vegetables may even carry lead residues from soil or air tainted by pesticides or pollution from incineration, factory emissions, car exhaust and burning waste oil. Paint chips and dust from lead-based insecticides also find their way into soil in backyards and sandboxes.

The Centers for Disease Control set the level of concern for youngsters at 10 micrograms per deciliter of blood (down from 25 micrograms per deciliter): research suggests that higher levels compromise physical and mental development. Lead accumulates over a lifetime, therefore people may be carrying deposits of this toxic chemical in their bones. Doctors claim that lead may reenter the bloodstream at any time as a result of severe biologic stress (pregnancy, menopause, prolonged immobilization and severe disease).

STATISTICS AND STUDIES

According to the EPA, 32 million Americans are drinking tap water that may be seriously contaminated with lead levels in excess of EPA guidelines. The media has been reporting water pollution for some time, but their focus as of late has been on drinking water contamination.

The EPA's first comprehensive test of municipal water supplies found that nearly 20 percent of the nation's largest cities have lead in drinking water in excess of the federally permissible levels. For example, it was reported that tap water in Syracuse, New York, has levels three times greater, and Utica, New York, six times greater than the EPA's lead "action level" of 15 parts per billion established in regulations under the Safe Drinking Water Act.

USA Today (January 19, 1993) looked at 200 homes in eight cities and found that Boston and Chicago had the most households with high levels of lead, with San Francisco, Washington, DC, and New York following behind. According to *US News & World Report*, July 29, 1991, lead levels at the tap in many New England cities, such as Providence, Rhode Island, Manchester, New Hampshire, and Boston, have been especially high because their "soft" (low mineral content) water is very effective at corroding pipes and allowing lead to invade the drinking water.

The government has been showing more involvement in the water issue. The EPA recently found water in homes served by 130 of the largest U.S. water supply systems had lead content exceeding federal health limits. Dr. Richard Maas of the University of North Carolina's Environmental Quality Institute reports that more than one-sixth of the nation's homes—17 percent—have faucets leaking high amounts of lead.

State Attorney General Dan Lungren of Sacramento, California, sued 16 of the nation's faucet manufacturers, saying their faucets are leaching enough lead into California's drinking water to potentially harm fetuses and children. Proposition 54, approved by California voters in 1986, requires companies to warn Californians if their products contain chemicals that, above certain levels, can cause cancer or birth defects. The law also forbids the discharging of these chemicals into drinking water or sources of drinking water. The lawsuit will force manufacturers to take action that they should have taken voluntarily years ago. The federal limit for lead in drinking water is 30 times higher than California standards.

The most publicized lead poisoning cases come from preschoolers ingesting paint chips. In Children's Hospital of Wisconsin in Milwaukee in 1990, Eric Rivera died of lead poisoning after consuming quantities of leaded paint chips, most likely over a period of time. Lead dust is less talked about, but equally as likely to be eaten by a child who constantly puts his or her fingers in the mouth.

Anne and Kevin Sheehan of Chatham, New York, bought an abandoned old house during her pregnancy with their third child. After the birth, the couple worked on the renovation during the evenings and weekends, taking every reasonable precaution. "We never had the kids in the house when we were sanding," says Anne. "And we always vacuumed afterward, which I now know is the worst thing because it spreads lead dust."

Last year she had her children tested for lead and discovered two-year-old Kate had a blood lead level of 29 micrograms; Kate had been exposed to lead since birth. The Sheehans had to move out of their home. Kate took oral chelating drugs for 12 weeks, which reduced her lead levels, but it's too early to know whether the youngster, now three, will suffer long-term damage.*

Less likely causes of lead poisoning are often overlooked, but they can be just as dangerous. In 1970 a California family suffered acute lead poisoning from drinking orange juice stored in a pitcher bought in Mexico. The Food and Drug Administration (FDA) subsequently set up requirements for testing pottery glazes on imports.

The Agency for Toxic Substances and Disease Registry estimates that between 3 and 4 million children suffer from exposure to lead at concentrations that place them at risk of adverse health effects.

DETECTION

The first step in the detection of surface lead (paint, dishware, solder) is to purchase an inexpensive lead stick kit. This is an easy-

*Good Housekeeping/Family Circle magazine.

to-use method in which the indicator changes color if lead is present. There are also home test kits available to detect lead in water. If any of these tests turn out to be positive, it is recommended that you contact a qualified lead inspector to identify the extent of the problem. You can call the EPA safe drinking water hotline for information on laboratories in your local area (800)426-4791.

SOLUTION

Lead paint should be a serious concern for any homeowner who lives in a house or apartment built before 1978. Have your home tested for lead. If the test is positive, consider removal of lead paint by professional contractors specializing in this area. Consult your state health or housing department for recommendations. Do not try to remove the lead paint yourself as the dust created can be more toxic than the paint.

Cover the area affected by lead paint with another surface: wallpaper, drywall, paneling, paint or nontoxic sealer (AFM). Never sand lead paint. If the surface is in need of sanding or removal of chipped paint, do not re-cover, but have it removed. If removal is not practical there are containment paints available that have been designed to cover lead paint. These paints, when dry, resemble a rubberized finish and are resilient. They are effective in containing any chipping and dusting of the old paint. Have carpets removed if lead dust contamination is suspected from interior or exterior sources, as they trap dust which cannot be removed through vacuuming.

If you find chipped lead paint, try to prevent any lead dust buildup by cleaning hard-surface floors with a wet mop rather than a broom, and wash windowsills and baseboards once a week with a trisodium phosphate cleaner. Place heavy furniture in front of painted windowsills and moldings and bushes next to any exterior lead paint in order to keep children away. If you suspect lead in the soil, plant grass to keep the dust down. If your child plays in a sandbox, make sure that you import clean sand to preclude lead ingestion from dirty fingers.

In order to safeguard yourself from lead in drinking water, run tap water at least 60 seconds prior to using it if the faucet has gone unused for more than six hours (lead settles out of solder and pipes). Use cold water for cooking or drinking. Lead does not leach as easily into cold water. An even better solution is to install NSF (not-for-profit product testing and certification organization) certified drinking water filters that remove lead (see chart: Water Contaminants, page 123) or remove pipes and replace with nonlead solder.

For protection against lead ingestion from food and drink, limit use of lead crystal ware, and avoid using lead dishes or pottery. Don't use older ceramic products unless they have been tested for lead coatings. Determine whether imported foods use lead soldered cans and eliminate them from your grocery cart. Also make sure that children get lots of iron and calcium in their diet. This will prevent the uptake of lead into the body. Regular meals also help, since more lead is absorbed on an empty stomach.

Be aware of children's toys containing lead. Many painted and assembled toys (especially imported ones) still may be contaminated. You may be able to use your stick test to identify them. It is absolutely essential that you do not let your children play with these toys.

If your child tests positive for lead poisoning at an acute level, there is help available. Chelation is a treatment that removes lead from the bloodstream. It is normally an intravenous method, although oral drugs are available. All children should be tested regularly. Contact your local or state health department for more information.

Good News

The government has been helping to reduce lead poisoning. The EPA Office of Drinking Water has proposed regulations under the Safe Drinking Water Act that establish a maximum contaminant level for lead in drinking water of five micrograms per liter and a maximum contaminant level goal of zero. In 1986 amendments to the Safe Drinking Water Act banned any further use of materials containing lead in public water supplies and in residences connected to public water supplies. In 1988 the U.S. Congress banned the use of lead-based solder in plumbing applications within homes and buildings. Lead levels in foods have dropped since most manufacturers stopped using leaded solder in cans.

Virtual elimination of lead from gasoline has decreased the deposition of lead on food crops and has been reflected in reductions in blood lead levels in children and adults.

A war is also being waged on lead paint. The U.S. Department of Housing and Urban Development now requires FHA borrowers purchasing homes built prior to 1978 to read and sign a lead-based paint disclosure notice. The notice must be signed before the sale may be consummated. This places the responsibility on the realtor to secure disclosure and acknowledgment.

In order to protect children during renovation, the Occupational Safety and Health Administration established standards regarding construction workers' handling of lead-based paints on site. The new standards are part of a mandate issued by Congress in 1992 in the National Housing Act's Residential Lead-Based Paint Hazard Reduction Act (Title 10).

With increased awareness and a pointed effort to reduce lead dust and lead in water, children will not have to suffer many of the consequences of lead poisoning. Further study should be undertaken by parents of young children.

On the following pages is a list of public water supplies that exceed lead action levels.

FOR MORE INFORMATION

"A Dish Owner's Guide to Potential Lead Hazards" (free), Environmental Defense Fund, 5655 College Avenue, Oakland, California 94618

EPA pamphlet, "Lead and Your Drinking Water," Consumer Products Safety Commission, 401 M Street, Washington, DC 20460

EPA Safe Drinking Water Hotline 1-800-426-4791

"Renovating Your Home Without Lead Poisoning Your Children" ($1, no cash), Conservation Law Foundation, Department L, 3 Joy Street, Boston, Massachusetts 02108

Public Water Supplies Exceeding Lead Action Levels
(standard is 15 parts per billion)

Location	Parts per billion
ARIZONA	
Phoenix	19
CALIFORNIA	
Palo Alto	18
San Francisco	30
CONNECTICUT	
Hartford	40
DISTRICT OF COLUMBIA	
Washington Aqueduct	18
FLORIDA	
Cocoa Beach	32
Daytona Beach	24
Escambia County	175
Fort Myers	34
Miami Beach	27
Pompano Beach	84
GEORGIA	
Douglasville	30
Gwinnett County	66
Macon-Bibb County	17
Marietta	22
North Fulton	53
Richmond County	48
Savannah	21
ILLINOIS	
Decatur	36
Evanston	25
Glenview	25
Oak Lawn	18
Oak Park	39
Waukegan	20
INDIANA	
Fort Wayne	21
Hammond	27

Location	Parts per billion
IOWA	
Cedar Rapids	80
Des Moines	21
MAINE	
Portland	70
MARYLAND	
Eldridge-Howard County	20
Potomac Plant	39
MASSACHUSETTS	
Boston Water and Sewer	48
Brookline Water Department	62
Framingham Water Division	100
Lowell Water Department	51
Newton Water Department	163
Somerville Water Department	84
Springfield	32
Waltham Water Division	52
Worcester Water Department	39
MICHIGAN	
Clinton Township	19
Dearborn	29
Detroit	21
Grand Rapids	35
Livonia	34
St. Clair Shores	23
Taylor	35
Warren	21
MINNESOTA	
Minneapolis	19
St. Paul	54

Location	Parts per billion
NEW HAMPSHIRE	
Nashua (Pennichuck)	45
NEW JERSEY	
Jersey City	84
Newark Water Department	27
Passaic Valley	24
Southeast Morris County	37
Trenton Water Department	18
Wayne Township	29
NEW YORK	
Binghamton	20
Elmira Water Board	20
Mount Vernon	62
New Rochelle Water	36
New York Aqueduct	55
Syracuse	50
Utica Board of Water	100
Yonkers	68
NORTH CAROLINA	
Asheville	29
Gastonia	17
OHIO	
Cleveland (Baldwin Plant)	25
(Crown Plant)	20
(Morgan)	19
(Nottingham)	25
OREGON	
Beaverton	28
Portland	41
PENNSYLVANIA	
Erie Bureau of Water	16
Lancaster	41
Lower Bucks County	37
Philadelphia Water Department	22

Location	Parts per billion
Plymouth Relief	31
Westmorland County (Beaver Run)	25
Westmorland County (Yough)	56
Williamsport	51
PUERTO RICO	
Fajardo Ceiba	60
Metropolitano	16
Rio Blan, Vieq	29
RHODE ISLAND	
Pawtucket	29
TEXAS	
Port Arthur	28
VIRGINIA	
Chesapeake	30
Portsmouth	26
Richmond	16
Occoquan-Woodbridge	22
WASHINGTON	
Alderwood Water Department	28
Bellevue	19
Bellingham Water Division	23
Northshore Utility	29
Seattle Water Department	19
Tacoma	32
WISCONSIN	
Madison Waterworks	16
Oshkosh Waterworks	17
Racine Waterworks	18
West Allis Waterworks	22

Water Systems News and Home Water Report, October, 1992.

MOLD

MOLD SPORES ARE everywhere. They grow in damp, cool places and become airborne travelers until they alight in places such as your nose or lungs.

DESCRIPTION

Molds (biological pollutants) are or were living organisms. They promote poor indoor air quality and may be a major cause of days lost from work or school and of doctor and hospital visits. Some can even damage surfaces inside and outside your home. Two conditions are essential to support mold growth: nutrients and moisture.

If your home exceeds the recommended 30 to 50 percent relative humidity, you may have a moisture problem. Humidity can be present in a home as a vapor (gas), liquid or solid. Air movement is the major water vapor transfer method and is the easiest method for intake into the body because mold attaches itself to moist particles.

Once mold spores attach themselves to you as a host, they can irritate your eyes, nose and throat, and cause shortness of breath, dizziness, lethargy, fever, digestive problems, humidifier fever, influenza, measles, chicken pox and other infectious diseases. Molds can trigger allergic reactions, including hypersensitivity pneumonitis, allergic rhinitis and some types of asthma. Many allergic reactions caused by biological allergens occur immediately after exposure; other allergic reactions are the result of previous exposures that you may be unaware of. As a result, people who have noticed only mild allergic reactions, or no reactions at all, may suddenly find themselves very sensitive to particular allergens.

A common place for mold to form is in the basement. This is due to excess moisture from washers or dryers in this area, and also from damp walls and stored items, such as newspapers, magazines, clothes, or stuffed furniture. In most basements which are even a little damp, spores are produced by the millions and eventually find their way into the house.

In warm or hot climates, humidity is normally handled through the use of dehumidifiers and air-conditioning. However, unless these appliances are cleaned frequently, mold can form in the moist areas within the units and be expelled into the air from the outflow. This airborne mold, depending on the type, can affect health if inhaled.

In colder climates, condensation can occur within the walls and on windows, creating a potential mold problem. Proper venting of moisture sources and use of indoor air-venting sources can help control the relative humidity.

Some cases of high relative humidity result from too many people or pets occupying a small space, as bodies generate moisture. A good rule of thumb is 250 square feet per person or pet. A family of four can produce up to four gallons of moisture per day within a home. High indoor relative humidity can cause significant building damage as well as health problems, such as respiratory troubles and diseases caused by microbial growth. Areas of high humidity can be created in the kitchen and bathroom from cooking without lids, heating or cooking with open-flame appliances, bathing or showering and hanging wet clothing and towels inside to dry. Aquariums and numerous houseplants can add to the moisture content indoors. Clothes dryers vented indoors can cause not only dust problems but excess moisture as well. Inadequate ventilation overall in a structure can add to moisture in the walls, attics and crawl spaces and cause prime breeding grounds for mold.

Faulty flame-fired appliances used for heating, water heating or cooking can be sources of moisture problems. Without adequate combustion air, these appliances can spill water vapor as well as deadly, odorless carbon monoxide gas into living space. You can identify incomplete combustion by an excessively yellow or wavy flame and windows that fog for no other reason.

Carpets can be a source of mold growth if the humidity level is high in the home or if the carpets have recently been cleaned and not allowed to dry thoroughly before humidity was introduced into the living area. Mold that forms in the backing of a carpet can remain and continue to promote spores because backing receives little air circulation and has a limited chance to dry out completely. It is prudent for homeowners to frequently inspect areas susceptible to dampness as mold and mildew are sometimes detectable by their scent and sometimes visible, although their spores—which travel through the air—are not.

Outdoor causes of excess moisture usually stem from improper drainage around foundations or from roof areas. Clay soil which limits absorption can channel water toward a house. This can cause seepage into the walls where moisture can breed mold and find its way into the living area. Checking for proper drainage and correcting any problems is the answer to reduction in this problem area.

STATISTICS AND STUDIES

Most information about sources and health effects of biological pollutants is based on studies of large office buildings and two surveys of homes in the northern United States and Canada. These surveys show that 30 to 50 percent of all structures have damp conditions which may encourage the growth and buildup of biological pollutants. This percentage will probably be higher in warm, moist climates, where an inordinate number of people are likely to develop allergies.

Larry Foster, president of Air Duct Decontamination, noticed 25 years ago that many of the men he was working with became ill during the cleaning of an industrial air-conditioning system. He removed some of the molds from the heating ducts and had them analyzed. They turned out to be penicillium and aspergillus, well known for causing allergic reactions and also implicated in such allergy-related diseases as hypersensitivity pneumonitis, allergic bronchopulmonary aspergillosis and eczema.

The following anecdote stresses the importance of cleaning potential mold sites. A woman suspected something was affecting her household when her grandchildren worked with her in the kitchen, where there was a large heating vent. They always felt sick and couldn't eat anything they had prepared. During the summer this woman developed symptoms which she attributed to her air conditioner. When she turned the heat on in the winter, she developed headaches and congested nasal passages, so she contacted the Atlanta Department of Health. They suggested that she have the ducts to her forced hot air system cleaned, which she did. The cleaners removed four to eight pounds of dust from the ducts. The next day she found that she did not need her antihistamine for the first time in a long time.

DETECTION

Use a humidistat to determine your home's humidity level. If you find over 50 percent humidity, follow the solutions offered to reduce moisture. Check visually for staining or fungus and use your sense of smell to identify musty odors which stem from a moldy condition.

Examine humidifiers and air conditioners, as they can produce lots of mold, especially if old water is left standing. Have dust from forced hot air ducts analyzed by a lab for possible biologicals or hire a duct-cleaning service to give you their opinion. Remember, they may just want to sell you their service. Mold collects in ducts after the summer season and becomes airborne when you fire up your heating system. This is a common reason why people get colds at the start of the heating season.

If you are highly allergic, contact a local lab to perform an on-site mold test for specific biologicals so you can identify the culprit and treat it properly.

SOLUTIONS

In order to wage war on mold, apply the following recommendations:

- Check and clean humidifiers and air conditioners often
- Check forced hot air ducts before heating season begins
- Check for outdoor drainage problems and eliminate them
- Eliminate roof leaks
- Eliminate plumbing leaks
- Vent clothes dryers to the outside
- Add a heat recovery ventilator to the living space for air circulation and moisture reduction
- Install bath and kitchen fans and run them during high moisture conditions or install an automatic timer on them to run at intervals
- Consider a dehumidifier for basements or high moisture areas
- Vent attic and crawl space properly; if you are unsure of procedures, call a local contractor
- If remodeling, add insulation and install vapor barrier between the inside wall and the insulation to prevent household moisture from collecting in the wall cavity
- Check for blocked furnace vents to promote venting of heating or cooking appliances
- Check length of flue to increase air draft of heating or cooking appliances
- Install an air cleaner unit that removes mold
- Check water trays under the refrigerator and clean if moldy
- Keep grout clean on any tiled areas
- Check wallpaper for signs of mold in the wallpaper paste; many pastes have antifungal additives, and although they control mold, they also off-gas toxic chemicals
- If using mold and mildew cleaners, be aware that commercial brands contain pesticides, formaldehyde, phenol, pentachlorophenol (restricted for outdoor use) and kerosene; a natural alternative is to mix borax or vinegar with water in

a spray bottle; several manufacturers of nontoxic products sell mildew removers

- To dry out a moldy area, put a portable heater in the room and let it bake the mold dry to a dust which can be wiped up.

Good News

Building scientists agree that homes should be built tightly and use a mechanical ventilation system to control moisture and air quality. Leaky houses deliver fresh air at an uneven rate depending on the wind outside, inside air temperature ratio and leak rate of the building. The air delivery is either excessive or insufficient, and has little to do with actual fresh air needs and moisture control of the house.

Energy conservation practices are aimed at trapping heated air indoors and reducing the infiltration of cold outside air. As a side effect of these practices, moisture is trapped indoors. The solution to excess humidity is a tightly constructed home and increased ventilation with the installation of heat recovery units.

Heat recovery ventilators (HRV's) are now being made by many manufacturers who are addressing the air quality control within homes and offices. Less expensive single units for smaller areas, and whole-house systems such as those manufactured by Honeywell, EZ Vent, VanEE, Vent Aire, AirExchange and Life-breath, are making it possible for home owners to have the best of both worlds: a tight house and adequate air ventilation and moisture control.

FOR MORE INFORMATION

Contact your local American Lung Association for copies of "Indoor Air Pollution Fact Sheets, Air Pollution in Your Home?" and U.S. Consumer Product Safety Commission, Washington, DC 20207 for "The Inside Story: A Guide to Indoor Air Quality and Humidifier Safety Alert."

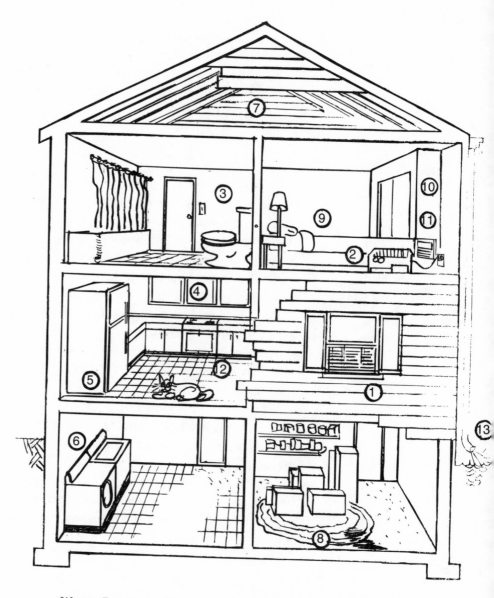

WHERE BIOLOGICAL POLLUTANTS MAY BE FOUND IN THE HOME

1. Dirty air conditioners
2. Dirty humidifiers and/or dehumidifiers
3. Bathroom without vents or windows
4. Kitchen without vents or windows
5. Dirty refrigerator drip pans
6. Laundry room with unvented dryer
7. Unventilated attic

8. Carpet on damp basement floor
9. Bedding
10. Closet on outside wall
11. Dirty heating/air-conditioning system
12. Dogs or cats
13. Water damage (around windows,
    the roof or the basement)

PESTICIDES

A FRIEND OF OURS had a brother who died from weed killer. He had a home in Brooklyn, New York, and fertilized his lawn every year with conventional fertilizer. The year he died, he used a fertilizer with weed killer in it and carefully took all the precautions listed in the instructions. One week later he began having severe leg pain that was slowly moving upward. His physician couldn't diagnose his illness and decided to take a wait-and-see approach since he wasn't incapacitated.

The man was employed as a sales representative. One day, as he approached a client's office, he fell over and died. The autopsy revealed that residue from the weed killer had penetrated all the protection he wore, entered his skin and destroyed most of his vital organs. This man followed the rules set by the manufacturer and still lost his life. A nontoxic alternative would have saved his life.

DESCRIPTION

Pesticides are chemicals used in and around the home to control weeds, insects, termites, rodents and fungi. They are sold as sprays, liquids, sticks, powder, crystals, balls and foggers or "bombs."

EPA surveys show that nine out of ten U.S. households use pesticides. One study reveals that 80 to 90 percent of most people's exposure to pesticides in the air occurs indoors. Measurable levels of up to a dozen pesticides have been found in the air inside

75

homes. Contamination can also occur through soil or dust that floats or is tracked in from outside, pesticides stored in containers and household surfaces that collect and then release pesticides.

Pesticides also have "inert" ingredients which are used to carry the active agent. Although nontoxic to the pest, they can be harmful to humans. For example, methylene chloride, a household product chemical, is an "inert."

Pesticides from aerial spraying in and around cropland may affect residents living downwind from a field. Pesticides applied from airplanes can drift as much as four miles, even with a no-wind condition.

Long-term exposure to pesticides can damage the liver, kidneys and lungs and cause paralysis, sterility, suppression of immune function, brain hemorrhages, decreased fertility and sexual function, heart problems and coma.

Symptoms arising from the use of pesticides include headaches, dizziness, muscle twitching, weakness, tingling, cough, breathing difficulties, depression, blurred vision, convulsions and nausea. The EPA is also concerned that the main ingredients in termiticides might cause long-term damage to the liver and central nervous system as well as increased risk of cancer.

Pesticides can end up in the food chain. The Canadian government found that 90 percent of our food already contains traces of pesticides. Children are more susceptible because their bodies are still forming. A report by the National Research Council recommends that the government set pesticide tolerance levels, which are the amounts of pesticides legally allowed on or in foods when they leave the farm. These regulations would take into account children's susceptibility and attempt to set acceptable levels of pesticide ingestion. Based on other information regarding health effects of pesticides, it seems that a no-pesticide level (in organically grown food) should be a target of every parent.

STATISTICS AND STUDIES

There are more than 34,000 pesticides, derived from about 600 basic chemical ingredients currently registered by the EPA for use in the United States. Pesticides are the number two cause of household poisonings in the United States. About 2.5 million children and adults are affected each year by such common household items as fly spray, ant and roach bait and insect repellents.

The most widely used weed killer in the world is 2,4D. It is still being manufactured even though it has been proven to have lethal effects on humans. During the Vietnam War tonnage of this chemical was used, with the result that Vietnamese babies were born with deformities. Veterans are now experiencing cancer and heart problems and some of their offspring have physical handicaps.

In 1986 the *Journal of the American Medical Association* reported the link between human cancer and exposure to 2,4D. A Harvard Medical School study verifies findings that show a single exposure to 2,4D can trigger changes in human brain activity that can cause loss of memory, depression, paranoia, irritability and other health problems. If you purchase weed killer, make sure it does not contain 2,4D.

Chlordane and three related termiticides, heptachlor, aldrin, and dieldrin, remain active for long periods of time; when airborne they last up to 30 years. Some insecticides, once applied, can never be removed. The only thing to do with a heavily fumigated house is move from it.

Approximately 91 percent of all American households apply about 300 million pounds of pesticides annually, including weed killer. Seventy percent of pesticide poisonings occur in children under five, and over half of those who die from pesticides are children. Many insecticides are relatively insoluble in water and are instead dispensed in petroleum-based solvents, to which a large number of individuals are sensitive. So not only are the principal (active) ingredients a potential source of trouble, but the carrier (or vehicle) may also cause problems.

Researchers at Hartford Hospital in Connecticut found that fatty breast tissue from women with malignant breast tumors contained more than twice as many PCB's (polychlorinated biphenyls) and DDE's (a by-product of the pesticide DDT) as the breast fat of women of the same age and weight who didn't have cancer. The study, which appeared in the *Archives of Environmental Health*, was conducted by a team of doctors led by

University of Michigan toxicologist Frank Falck. Dr. Falck believes most of the women in his study were exposed to the chemicals in their diets rather than in industrial jobs or in other environmental contexts.

Poison control centers are unable to obtain information from manufacturers as to the makeup of "inert" ingredients in pesticides. The EPA has a list of some possibly inert ingredients, 28 of which are suspected carcinogens. Xylene, a popular one, is known to be used in 2,216 pesticide products. Chlordane has a half-life of 50 years. The EPA banned this substance from termite pesticides and the ruling was subsequently overturned. In 1980 the agency successfully banned it again.

DDT and other pesticides have been used on many commercial aircraft arriving at foreign locations to control transfer of pests and disease. The techniques for control include spraying the cabin of the aircraft with passengers still in their seats, prior to disembarkment. Chemical sensitivities and the health of the passengers have not been considered until recently and not in all countries.

If you are sensitive to pesticides, ask your airline whether it employs this procedure and determine whether there are any alternatives or precautions you can take.

DETECTION

If you suspect a high concentration of pesticides in your home, contact a local laboratory and have an air or dust test performed. Water analysis also can indicate residual pesticides which have filtered down into groundwater. This is most common in agricultural areas.

SOLUTIONS

Don't use pesticides! Investigate the Integrated Pest Management (IPM) methods or purchase natural pest control products from companies and catalogues such as *Gardens Alive* (812)537-

8650. The goal of IPM programs is to combat insects and diseases with a combination of biological controls and other methods which are as undisruptive to the environment as possible, especially using natural enemies of the pests. If you decide to use pesticides, read the label. It is against the law to use any pesticide in a manner inconsistent with the directions.

Contract with a chemical-free pesticide company to rid your house of pests. The proven methods that will not endanger your health are microwave, heat treatment, electrogun, liquid nitrogen, borax treatment for wood and nematodes and diatomaceous earth for outside use.

Never use no-pest strips to kill bugs, especially in the nursery, as most contain harmful chemicals that can out-gas and affect your baby's health.

Beware of carpets, wallpaper and wallpaper paste treated with insecticides. There are nontoxic substitutes available from Environmental Construction Outfitters, 1-800-238-5008.

Good News

Governments have entered into pesticide regulation. Since October, 1977, the EPA has required laboratory safety tests at the manufacturer's expense before any new pesticide is allowed on the market. Included must be tests for acute-exposure effects and the lethal dose in animals, and chronic-exposure tests for cancer, genetic mutation, birth defects and fertility. All pesticides legally sold in the United States must bear an EPA-approved label to show that they are registered.

In 1990 the Canadian government proposed setting a legal tolerance level of 20 parts per trillion of dioxin in food. This was deemed necessary because most food contains traces of this pesticide.

Pennsylvania state legislators, urged by the environmental group Clean Water Action, are working to enact the Pesticide Notification Act in both state legislatures. The bills would require schools to exhaust all nontoxic pest control methods before turning to chemicals, which must be applied at least 24 hours before students enter a building, and to make these treatments known to parents and teachers beforehand.

The termiticides aldrin and dieldrin have been banned and

chlordane and heptachlor cannot be used until an application method that will not result in any measurable exposure to household occupants is successfully developed.

IPM coordinates use of pest control methods, taking advantage of all methods, including nontoxic ones. The EPA encourages the IPM approach and is working with school officials and others to develop IPM in schools.

Linda and Bill Bonvie, in an *Earth Journal* article of Nov./Dec. 1993 entitled "Flying in the Mist," had news for domestic U.S. air travelers: A 1983 memo from Assistant Surgeon General Donald R. Hopkins regarding the Centers for Disease Control position on insect control in international sea and air travel notes that "the U.S. cannot support the use of insecticides in aircraft areas with passengers present. Pesticides registered for such use should not be inhaled." In effect, the safety issue precludes a U.S. requirement for disinfection. This protects passengers flying into and throughout the United States from pesticide spraying, but there is no such protection for Americans leaving the country, even on American-owned airlines, which must comply with World Health Organization guidelines and destination country regulations.

FOR MORE INFORMATION:

Bio-Integral Resource Center, P.O. Box 7414, Berkeley, CA 94707, for least toxic method of pest management

BIRC booklets on termites (510) 524-2567

Blizzard System (liquid nitrogen) (213) 422-1131

"Citizen's Guide to Pesticides," R. Woods Consumer Information Center (50 cents), 142 W Pueblo, Pueblo, CO 81009

Electro-gun extermination: call for local technician, 1-800-543-5651

Environmental Health Coalition Fact Sheet. (619) 235-0281, information on safer flea control for pets

Integrated Pest Management, Field Operations Division Program Communications Branch (703) 557-5076

Isothermics (heat tents) (714) 974-0951

National Pesticide Telecommunications Network, 1-800-858-PEST

Northwest Coalition for Alternatives to Pesticides, P.O. Box 1393, Eugene, OR 97440

Taunton Press, Box 5506, Newtown, CT 06470, for "Common Sense Pest Control"

RADON

DESCRIPTION

ABOUT ONE OUT OF every 15 homes in the United States is estimated to have elevated radon levels. It can be a problem in schools and workplaces too. The only known health effect associated with exposure to elevated levels of radon is lung cancer. The EPA estimates that about 5,000 to 20,000 lung cancer deaths a year in the United States may be attributable to radon. The American Cancer Society estimates there is a total of about 139,000 lung cancer deaths from all causes (1988 figures).

Radon is a colorless, odorless, tasteless gas that occurs worldwide in the environment as a by-product of the natural decay of uranium present in the earth. It is present in varying quantities in the atmosphere and in soils around the world. Radon is estimated to cause many thousands of lung cancer deaths each year. In fact, the surgeon general has warned that radon is the second leading cause of lung cancer in the United States.

Radon gas breaks down into radioactive particles that remain in the air. As you breathe these particles, they can become trapped in your lungs. As these particles continue to break down, they release bursts of energy (radiation) that can damage lung tissue.

Only smoking causes more lung cancer deaths than radon. If you smoke and your home has high radon levels, your risk of lung cancer is especially high.

Radon that is present in surrounding soil or in well water can be a source of radon in a home. Air pressure inside your home is usually lower than pressure in the soil around your home's foundation. Because of this difference in pressure, your house acts like a vacuum, drawing radon in through foundation cracks and other openings. It can enter through cracks in solid floors, construction joints, cracks in walls, gaps in suspended floors, gaps around service pipes, cavities inside walls and water supply.

Radon may also be present in well water and can be released into the air in your home when water is used for showering and other household purposes. In most cases, radon entering a home through water is a small risk compared with radon entering a home from soils. In a small number of homes, building materials, such as cement floors and foundations made with radon-containing soil, can give off radon.

The concentration of radon in air is measured in units of picocuries per liter (pCi/L) of air. Estimates suggest that most homes will contain from one to two pCi of radon per liter of air. If preliminary tests indicate radon levels greater than 4 pCi/L of air in livable areas of a home, a follow-up test is recommended. The EPA estimates that indoor radon levels will increase by about 1 pCi/L of air for every 10,000 pCi/L of radon in water if radon is found in water through proper testing methods.

The national average level of radon in homes is estimated to be 1½ pCi/L, but in some cases levels in homes have been found as high as 200 pCi/L. With effective remediation techniques, these levels can be reduced to 4 pCi/L of air and sometimes less.

STATISTICS AND STUDIES

The EPA has determined that short-term exposure to a high concentration of radon is not as severe a risk as long-term exposure to a lower level of the gas. This is based on the EPA's risk assessments assuming an individual is exposed to a given concentration of radon over a lifetime of roughly 70 years and spends 75 percent of his or her time in the home. Because it takes 1,602 years for only half the radon atoms to disintegrate, radon molecules tend to accumulate over time, causing concentrations to become higher.

The EPA estimates that the risk of dying from lung cancer as the result of an annual radon level of 5 picocuries is equivalent to the risk from smoking 10 cigarettes a day or having 200 chest x rays a year. The National Academy of Sciences estimates the risk as up to ten times higher for smokers, partially because radon can hitch a ride directly into the lungs on tobacco particles that remain suspended in smoke.

Unlike potential cancer sources such as many chemicals, radon is particularly dangerous because it is known, not merely suspected, to be a carcinogen in humans. In homes where it exists at high levels, people tend to receive more exposure than they do to many other possible carcinogens. That's because people spend so much time at home.

In 1988 the surgeon general issued a National Public Health Advisory warning the public about the risks associated with exposure to elevated levels of radon. The advisory recommended that most homes be tested, even if an adjacent home is radon free. One man absorbed so much radiation from the radon in his home that he set off the radiation alarm when he entered a nuclear power plant. Yet his neighbor's house had no radon at all. This illustrates the specific nature of radon. If you live in one of the estimated 6 million American homes with high radon levels, you needn't panic. The effects of radon take place over many years, but you should begin mitigation immediately.

In a study of schools in 16 states, 19 percent of the 3,000 rooms tested had readings above EPA's action level of 4 pCi/L. The highest level found was 135 pCi/L, the equivalent of having over 10,000 chest x rays per year. Workplaces also can have radon hazards which compromise workers spending considerable time in one location. Homes and schools with high levels of radon can affect children, who are even more vulnerable because they breathe faster and, as they grow, their rapidly dividing cells may be more susceptible to radiation damage.

DETECTION

Two types of radon detectors are most commonly used in homes: charcoal canisters that are exposed for two to seven days;

and alpha track detectors that are exposed for one month or longer.

You can use a testing device or company that is state certified and/or listed in EPA's Radon Measurement Proficiency Program, or purchase home radon tests kits from hardware stores, eco stores, catalogues or local laboratories. If your test results indicate a radon level of 4 pCi/L or more, contact your state radon office for a list of certified labs close to you and have a second test performed (phone numbers listed below).

SOLUTIONS

It is suggested that you use a contractor trained to fix radon problems. EPA's Radon Contractor Proficiency (RCP) Program requires contractors to take training courses and pass an exam before being listed in EPA's National RCP Report.

If your house is set on a slab, your contractor can use the following radon reduction methods: subslab suction, drain tile suction, sump hole suction or block wall suction. Active subslab suction is the most common method. Suction pipes are inserted through the floor slab into the crushed rock or soil underneath. They may also be inserted below the concrete slab from outside the house. Acting like a vacuum cleaner, a fan connected to the pipes draws the radon gas from below the house and then releases it into the outdoor air. Passive subslab suction is similar except that it relies on air currents instead of a fan. For crawl spaces, radon levels can sometimes be lowered by ventilating the crawl space passively or with the use of a fan. The submembrane depressurization method sucks the air from beneath a layer of plastic laid on the soil.

For basements it is important to seal cracks and other openings in the foundation. The EPA does not recommend the use of sealing alone to reduce radon because, by itself, sealing has not been shown to lower radon levels significantly or consistently.

For air circulation methods which prevent radon buildup, install a fan to blow air into the basement or living area from either upstairs or outdoors. This attempts to create enough pressure at the lowest level indoors to prevent radon from entering the house. Natural ventilation is a temporary radon reduction technique as it helps only while windows are open. Heat recovery ventilators (air-to-air heat exchangers) can be installed to increase ventilation. These units prewarm fresh incoming air with the exiting stale air. There could be increased heating or cooling costs with HRV's but not as great as ventilation without heat recovery.

After your contractor has performed mitigation procedures, have him or her install a radon warning device after systems are in place to monitor operation and effectiveness.

If you have radon in your water, a simple activated carbon water filter can be installed to absorb it. These can be purchased from catalogues, eco stores, hardware and lumber outlets and water appliance dealers.

Good News

The federal government has undertaken an extensive public outreach effort to encourage individuals to test their homes. This effort includes a national hotline, 1-800-SOS-RADON, for obtaining further information on radon testing.

The EPA is working closely with state and local governments and the private sector to research and demonstrate cost-effective methods for reducing indoor radon levels, and with builders to develop radon-resistant new construction techniques. The agency has also established a national Radon Contractor Proficiency (RCP) Program that evaluates a contractor's ability to fix radon problems in residences. The RCP list is available from state radiation offices.

A state may make funds available to schools and local governments to develop public information materials, conduct radon surveys of schools, establish mitigation demonstration programs and conduct training activities. This is part of a program established by the EPA to enhance state radon programs.

FOR MORE INFORMATION:

EPA Drinking Water Hotline 1-800-426-4791
Government Hotline 1-800-SOS-RADON

•Brochures:
"A Citizen's Guide to Radon, Radon Reduction Methods (A Homeowner's Guide), The Inside Story—A Guide to Indoor Air Quality," EPA, Public Information Center, 401 M Street SW, Washington, DC 20460

"Consumer's Guide to Radon Reduction," EPA, Superintendent of Documents, U.S. Government Printing Office, Mail Stop SSOP, Washington, DC 20402-9328

"Radon Reduction Methods," R. Woods Consumer Information Center, Department 170, 142 W Pueblo, Pueblo, CO 81009

"Radon in Schools," National Education Association and National Parent Teacher Association, EPA 1-800-SOS-RADON

State Radon Offices

ALABAMA	(205) 261-5315
ALASKA	(907) 465-3019
ARIZONA	(602) 255-4845
ARKANSAS	(501) 661-2301
CALIFORNIA	(415) 540-2134
COLORADO	(303) 331-4812
CONNECTICUT	(203) 566-3122
DELAWARE	1-800-554-4636
DISTRICT OF COLUMBIA	(202) 727-7728
FLORIDA	1-800-543-8279
GEORGIA	(404) 894-6644
HAWAII	(808) 548-4383
IDAHO	(208) 334-5933
ILLINOIS	(217) 786-6384
INDIANA	1-800-272-9723
IOWA	(515) 281-7781
KANSAS	(913) 296-1560
KENTUCKY	(502) 564-3700

State Radon Offices

LOUISIANA	(504) 925-4518
MAINE	(207) 289-3826
MARYLAND	1-800-872-3666
MASSACHUSETTS	(413) 586-7525
MICHIGAN	(517) 335-8190
MINNESOTA	(612) 623-5341
MISSISSIPPI	(601) 354-6657
MISSOURI	1-800-669-7236
MONTANA	(406) 444-3671
NEBRASKA	(402) 471-2168
NEVADA	(702) 885-5394
NEW HAMPSHIRE	(603) 271-4674
NEW JERSEY	1-800-648-0394
NEW MEXICO	(505) 827-2940
NEW YORK	1-800-458-1158
NORTH CAROLINA	(919) 733-4283
NORTH DAKOTA	(701) 224-2348
OHIO	1-800-523-4439
OKLAHOMA	(405) 271-5221
OREGON	(503) 229-5797
PENNSYLVANIA	1-800-23-RADON
PUERTO RICO	(809) 767-3563
RHODE ISLAND	(401) 277-2438
SOUTH CAROLINA	(803) 734-4631
SOUTH DAKOTA	(605) 773-3153
TENNESSEE	(615) 741-4634
TEXAS	(512) 835-7000
UTAH	(801) 538-6734
VERMONT	(802) 828-2886
VIRGINIA	1-800-468-0138
VIRGIN ISLANDS	(809) 774-3320
WASHINGTON	1-800-323-9727
WEST VIRGINIA	(304) 348-3526
WISCONSIN	(608) 273-5180
WYOMING	(307) 777-7956

Radon Equivalent
To X-rays per year

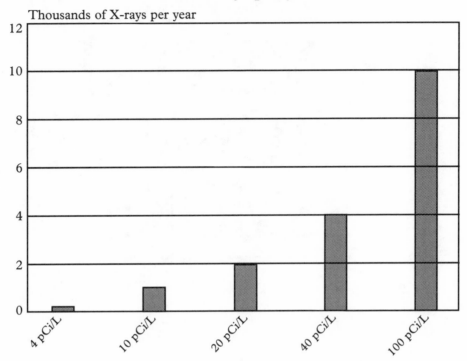

ENVIRON-MENTAL TOBACCO SMOKE

DESCRIPTION

NOT TOO MUCH will be said here about tobacco smoke because most of us have been educated on the subject through the print and television media. However, passive smoke, that caused by the burning tobacco product and exhaled by the smoker, will be covered.

This smoke is a complex mixture of 4,700 compounds, including both gases and particles (see section on combustion gases). It can have the following health effects: eye, nose and throat irritation; headaches; bronchitis; pneumonia; increased risk of ear and respiratory infections in children; lung cancer; and heart disease.

90

STATISTICS AND STUDIES

Environmental tobacco smoke gives off benzene, a known carcinogen. Long-term exposure to hydrogen cyanide, another component of tobacco smoke, is considered dangerous at levels of about 10 ppm; the concentration in cigarette smoke is 1,600 ppm. Studies indicate that exposure to tobacco smoke may increase the risk of lung cancer by an average of 30 percent in nonsmoking spouses of smokers. Very young children exposed to smoking at home are more likely to be hospitalized for bronchitis and pneumonia. Recent studies suggest that environmental tobacco smoke may also contribute to heart disease.

The 1986 surgeon general's report concluded that physical separation of smokers and nonsmokers in a common air space, such as different rooms within the same house, may reduce, but not eliminate, nonsmokers' exposure to environmental tobacco smoke. Natural or mechanical ventilation techniques do not remove these pollutants from home air as quickly as they build up because smoking produces such large amounts of them.

DETECTION

Tobacco smoke is easily detected by smell or sight, but if you need positive identification, install a passive cigarette detector—a disklike tester similar to a carbon monoxide detector. These detectors are available from laboratories, catalogues, and eco stores.

SOLUTIONS

Do not let anyone smoke in your home or building, but if that is not possible, install air purification devices and/or heat recovery ventilators to help reduce the effects.

Do not frequent places of business or entertainment where smoking is allowed, and do not permit young children to be exposed to cigarette smoke.

Good News

Smoking is banned on airplane flights in the United States over a certain length of time, and for some airlines, on all flights. It is also banned in many businesses and public areas.

Many restaurants have installed air filtration and air exchange systems in their dining rooms to reduce effects from smoking in designated areas.

During World War II, the Atomic Energy Commission developed high-efficiency particulate arrestance (HEPA) filters to remove radioactive dust from industrial exhausts. These filters are good for particles down to .3 microns in size and are rated at 99.9 percent efficiency. Tobacco smoke falls into this category and installation of this type of filter can help in passive tobacco smoke particle reduction. Activated carbon air filtration is successful in reducing tobacco smoke gases. Both the HEPA filter and activated carbon systems are available in a variety of air filtration units suitable to home use.

FOR MORE INFORMATION

Contact local chapters of the American Lung Association.

VOLATILE ORGANIC COMPOUNDS

A REPORT WAS RECEIVED regarding a Canadian teenager who, although she was very athletic during her school years, became disabled and was in and out of a wheelchair. Her symptoms included severe pain and weakness in her legs, chronic fatigue, lack of concentration and seizures. She was diagnosed as having a variant of multiple sclerosis or a psychosomatic condition. The diagnosis was uncertain.

When she was 19, the girl decided to follow a course of treatment for chemical sensitivities similar to that used in the Environmental Health Clinic in Dallas, Texas. By the sixth week her pains has subsided, her seizures stopped and she was able to walk a mile and a half a day. She is now able to resume a near normal life, but any contact with volatile chemicals causes an immediate onset of symptoms. She was wise enough to seek out information on environmental illness and lucky to have found a program that works.

DESCRIPTION

Other stories can illustrate the scope of symptoms that can occur because of exposure to volatile organic compounds. People may be exposed to many substances for years without a reaction until a specific incidence triggers symptoms. This intolerance can last a lifetime. A worker in a packaging company complained of lethargy, weakness, light-headedness, headaches, difficulty in concentrating, decreased mental activity, loss of visual acuity with difficulty in focusing, nausea, anorexia and increased tolerance to chemical odors. Prior to these symptoms, he had been in good health. It was discovered that his company recently began packaging a concentrated room deodorant.

During the process, some of the contents spilled, saturating the wooden floor over which the worker breathed during the next five months. He not only developed a reaction to the chemicals in the deodorant, but to all chemicals of petroleum origin, the main offender in the deodorant. These included perfumes, floor wax, and artificial food dyes and pesticide residues, which are found in many foods.

Volatile organic compounds (VOC's) are chemically unstable—although they may be liquid or solid, they readily vaporize or turn into gas. They also combine with other chemicals to create compounds that may cause toxic reactions when inhaled or absorbed through the skin.

The ability of organic compounds to influence health varies from producing minor discomfort to producing chronic disease. Many are suspected carcinogens. Side effects include eye and respiratory tract irritation, headaches, dizziness, visual disorders, memory impairment, depression, kidney problems, migraines, nervous system damage, wheezing and asthma. In addition to health hazards, VOC's can affect the atmosphere, contributing to smog and ground-level ozone pollution.

The presence of toxic vapors is more difficult to recognize than respirable particles, and on the average potentially more dangerous. One reason is that vapors penetrate the body's filtering system with ease—past the nose hairs, over the sticky bronchial substances, across the tracheal cilia, right into the alveoli, the minute sacs deep in the lungs where the exchange of carbon dioxide and oxygen in the blood takes place. Here they can pass easily through the permeable membranes and enter the bloodstream to be carried to all parts of the body. Vapors can go undetected unless they are identified by the sense of smell. Our body reacts to smells such as ammonia, and we should all be alerted to these reactions as warnings.

Often a person who simply dislikes particular smells is subsequently found to have been reacting physically to them. Interestingly, many people who state that they like certain odors also are adversely affected by them, particularly if exposed to the vapors regularly. Here the adaptation syndrome is in effect; the individual has become used to inhaling the vapors, and even though he or she is reacting badly to them on a long-term basis, the immediate response is pleasure.

Organic compounds (solvents) are widely used as ingredients in household products because of their many useful characteristics, such as the ability to dissolve substances and evaporate quickly. Paints, varnishes and wax all contain organic solvents, as do many cleaning, disinfecting, cosmetic, degreasing and hobby products, moth repellents, air fresheners and aerosol sprays. Stored fuels also release organic chemicals. All of these products can release organic compounds while you are using them, and to some degree, when they are stored. Some of the more common compounds are discussed here.

Benzene is a known human carcinogen. The main indoor sources are environmental tobacco smoke, stored fuel and paint supplies and automobile emissions in attached garages. Benzene has been linked as a causative agent to leukemia since 1928.

Perchloroethylene is the chemical most widely used in dry cleaning. In laboratory studies it has been shown to cause cancer in animals. Recent studies indicate that people breathe low levels of this chemical in homes where dry cleaned goods are stored and when they wear dry-cleaned clothing.

Methylene chloride is known to cause cancer in animals. It is converted to carbon monoxide in the body and causes symptoms associated with exposure to carbon monoxide. It is usually found in paint strippers, adhesive removers, aerosol spray paints and pesticide bombs.

Most *stains*, *varnishes* and *sealers* contain acetone, lead, methanol and pentachlorophenol, styrene, toluene and benzene. Polyurethane wood finishes contain 2-ethoxyethanol, which causes a chronic toxicity that builds up until a limit is reached. The distinctive smell of paint is actually dibutyl and diethyl phthalate and a host of other compounds that cause nausea, dizziness and severe headaches.*

Adhesives and *glue* may contain acetaldehyde, acetone, formaldehyde, dibutyl and diethyl phthalates, methanol, methyl and ethyl ketone, methylene chloride, phenol and xylenes.*

Furniture strippers, *furniture*, and *wall coverings* can contain acetone, methyl ethyl ketone, methylene chloride, toluene and xylenes.*

All-purpose cleaners can harbor fumes from ammonia, chlorine and cresol.*

STATISTICS AND STUDIES

EPA research has found that a dozen common organic pollutants are two to five times higher inside homes than outside, regardless of whether the homes are in the city or the country. They also found that not only are these compounds toxic while an individual is using them, but they can persist in the air long after the activity is completed. During and for several hours immediately after certain activities, such as paint stripping, levels may be a thousand times greater than outdoor levels.

The EPA has also listed fumes from slightly damp dry-cleaned items as a common indoor air pollutant. Ingredients may include perchloroethylene, benzene, chlorine, formaldehyde, naphthalene, toluene, trichloroethylene and xylene.

Cleaning products can cause a wide variety of health problems—from a simple skin rash obtained while washing dishes, or burning eyes from a whiff of ammonia, to death from acci-

*Information on the above products and associated toxins is provided by American Formulating and Manufacturing (AFM), makers of products for the chemically sensitive (619) 239-0321.

dental ingestion of drain cleaner. Despite the fact that labels on nearly all cleaning products clearly state "Keep Out of Reach of Children," accidental poisonings occur frequently, especially among infants and children who cannot read the warnings. Many of these products also give off volatile hazardous fumes. Not only is one exposed to them during use, but they stay trapped inside a home until they can escape through an open window.

Plastics out-gas many toxic chemicals. The National Aeronautics and Space Administration found polyester to be the synthetic material that released the most fumes. Acrylonitrile (Lucite/Plexiglas) is a suspected human carcinogen, as are epoxy resins, polyvinyl chloride (PVC), polyvinylpyrrolidone (PVP), found in some hairsprays, and polyethylene.

Nylon can cause reactions as both benzene and phenol are used in the manufacturing process and may linger in the material. Tetrafluoroethylene (Teflon) can cause irritation owing to producing small amounts of poisonous gases when heated. Hard plastics (Formica, etc) do not outgas for long periods of time, as do soft plastics.

In 1977 researchers from the National Institute for Occupational Safety and Health conducted tests with a standard paint remover containing 52 percent benzene. In a two-car garage, they stripped the paint from an end table while measuring the fumes. They found that a person exposed for five minutes would inhale more than 43 times the amount permitted by federal occupational exposure standards.

The researchers concluded that until regulatory action is taken by appropriate government agencies, or voluntary action is taken by responsible industries, concerned citizens must take action to protect themselves. Unfortunately, little information is being distributed to the consumer on the hazards of products containing VOC's.

DETECTION

If you think you have an outgassing problem from a newly decorated or constructed building, contact a laboratory to perform a

VOC test. Read labels on all household products, cleaners and decorating items. This may not help unless you are familiar with the "big" words listed as ingredients, but if you recognize any of those listed in the last section . . . beware! Use your sense of smell to alert you to possible toxins during application of these products.

SOLUTIONS

Minimize your use of organic solvent-based floor finishes, paints, stains or adhesives, but if you cannot find a substitute, test small amounts by smell or on your skin for immediate reactions before using these products in quantity.

Investigate using alternatives to toxic paints, adhesives and varnishes, but if you must use them, apply a finish coat with a nontoxic sealant in order to prevent outgassing. Buy household products in small quantities, and dispose of (with proper hazardous waste methods) unused or little-used containers. Avoid storing waxes, floor strippers, cleaners and paints in plastic containers (vapors can pass right through them) in confined places such as the cabinet under the sink, where vapors can build up to dangerous levels.

Provide for maximum ventilation during painting. If you have an exhaust fan, have it run continuously while applying VOC-based products. Consider purchasing an air filtration unit to absorb VOC's after the finish work is completed; as a permanent measure, consider installation of a heat recovery ventilator (see section on clean air) to reduce any residual effects of VOC's.

Do not pick up dry cleaning (which normally uses VOC chemicals) if it has a strong odor. Wait until it has been properly dried and air out dry-cleaned clothes before wearing them. Investigate the new establishments that use environmentally friendly cleaning methods.

Find alternatives to pesticide bombs, especially those with methylene chloride. There are many safe pest management methods available with products offered from catalogues such as *Gardens Alive*, (812) 537-8650.

Investigate household chemicals used in your cleaning, cosmetic and hobby products and substitute with nontoxic alternatives such as those listed in *Nontoxic, Natural and Earthwise* by

Debra Lynn Dadd. Even shoe polish can be harmful, therefore it is best used outdoors.

Good News

Many state regulations now require or recommend reduced levels of VOC's in paint; these levels should appear on the label. Many manufacturers of paints, adhesives and solvents are producing low VOC products or nontoxic alternatives. For a listing of those companies, contact Environmental Construction Outfitters, 1-800-238-5008.

Dry cleaners now have methods to recapture perchloroethylene during the dry cleaning process. They can save money by reusing it and remove more of the chemical during the pressing and finishing processes (some do a better job at removing this chemical than others.)

A process called Sorbathene was designed to remove 99.9 percent of volatile organic chemicals from vent streams during manufacturing. The method was developed by AWD Technologies of Rockville, Maryland, a hazardous waste management and remediation company and subsidiary of Dow Chemical. In contrast with other technologies, Sorbathene employs an adsorption process to capture the chemicals for recycling. It can be used to reduce emissions from truck terminals, marine terminals and production plants, according to AWD.

FOR MORE INFORMATION

Annie Berthold-Bond, *Clean & Green: The Complete Guide to Nontoxic and Environmentally Safe Household Cleaning*, Woodstock, N.Y.: Ceres Press, 1990

Consumer Product Safety Hotline 1-800-638-CPSC

Household Hazardous Waste: A Bibliography of Useful References and List of State Experts, EPA, RCRA/Superfund Hotline 1-800-424-9346

Massachusetts League of Women Voters, 8 Winter Street, Boston MA 02108, for setting up for hazardous waste collections in your town

Toxic Substance Control Act Information Service (202) 554-1404

SYNTHETIC CARPET

In 1989 a Baltimore lighting store owner installed new carpet as part of his renovation. Shortly thereafter his sales clerk, his wife and son, and even vendors, began to complain of chest pains, headaches, sore throats, slurred speech, dizziness and forgetfulness. The owner moved to a new location and installed new carpeting, but still the symptoms persisted. He and his wife, even though no longer in that business, have developed chemical sensitivities to other substances as well.

The store owner sent his carpet to a lab for analysis; this resulted in test mice either developing identical symptoms or dying when exposed to air from the carpet sample. The lab suspected the chemical 4-phenylcyclohexene or 4-PC (a by-product of styrene and butadiene), the latex adhesive that holds carpet fibers to backing. Also, it was suspected that 4-PC interacting with other chemicals in the carpet could combine to produce other toxins.

In 1980 a Kentucky home owner installed new carpet and noticed that the spiders that normally crawled throughout the house became immobilized on the new flooring. The home owner and his family gradually developed health symptoms and decided to have the carpet tested. Chemicals found in the carpet were ethylbenzene, formaldehyde, methacrylic acid, toluene, amine and styrene. When the carpet was removed, the spiders came back. The family's symptoms lessened, but they had developed hypersensitivities to other irritants because of the continuous chemical attack from carpet outgassing.

CBS television has aired a segment showing mice dying after exposure to the chemicals in carpet, and much publicity has surrounded the story about workers at a Florida office who became ill following new carpet installation. Carpets, especially older ones, can harbor microbiological contaminants and the chemicals that out-gas from them have been implicated in several lawsuits by people who developed illnesses after installing new carpets.

Synthetic carpeting can add to indoor air pollution owing to the out-gassing of volatile chemicals from the carpeting and the chemicals used in adding stain-resistant coverings and fungicides. It is important to remember that carpet is part of a total floor covering system that may include the cushion and installation adhesives, also potential sources of emissions.

When new carpet is installed, it may produce an odor. All such odors are caused by chemicals. However, some people are more sensitive to these odors than others. Some of the chemicals that carpets off-gas are formaldehyde, xylene, and ethylbenzene. These and other chemicals, according to some indoor-air experts, can make sensitive occupants experience flulike symptoms or even cause permanent illness. Formaldehyde is used in manufacturing carpet because it is the least expensive bonding compound. However, it may also be the most expensive ingredient because of the potential health problems it creates.

Symptoms from these chemicals can be as diverse as burning eyes, memory problems, chills and fever, sore throats, joint pain, chest tightness, cough, numbness, nausea, dizziness, lightheadedness, blurred or double vision, nervousness, depression and difficulty in concentrating.

If your carpet is over five years old, the chances of toxic reactions are minimal, as most of the fungicides and other chemicals have gassed out. However, the carpeting then becomes a breeding ground for dust mites and mold. This is especially hazardous in schools, where diseases are easily spread.

STATISTICS

In October, 1987, the EPA installed 27,000 square yards of new carpet in their Waterside Mall office complex in Washington, D.C. By January, health problems began showing up among employees. Eighteen months later, an official EPA statement indicated that although the agency was unable to establish any scientific link between the carpet and employees' symptoms, it removed the carpet in areas of high employee complaints. EPA employees made their own analysis of the air quality data.

Based on information from a 1987 University of Arizona study that isolated the chemical compound 4-PC from carpeting, the employees began to monitor this chemical and found it to be the culprit. It is a by-product of the process used to make the latex backing for carpets. While the carpeting industry claims that animal tests show 4-PC to be harmless, an EPA risk-assessment group predicted that it could create nervous system and genetic problems.

Levels of 4-PC of up to 20 parts per billion (ppb) have been measured in new carpet. Four days after installation, levels fall to about 10 ppb, and after two months decrease to 1 to 2 ppb. You can smell 4-PC at a minimum level of .5 ppb. According to the Carpet Manufacturing Association, limited research has found no link between adverse health effects and the levels of chemicals emitted by new carpet.

Some people report allergy or flulike symptoms that they believe are caused by newly installed carpet; however, such symptoms could also be attributed to other sources. Anderson Labs, specialists in the health effects of indoor air who were interviewed in the CBS carpet segment, found in tests that some batches of carpet cause chemically related illness in mice and others do not. They advise not using carpets in schools, especially where children are close to the floor.

DETECTION

Unless your carpet is wool, cotton or one of the new low-toxic nylon types, suspect synthetic carpeting. Almost all wall-to-wall carpeting is of the chemical variety. If you suspect an out-gassing problem, send a sample to a lab or to the Carpet and Rug Institute (CRI) (see below). If your carpet is five years old, don't worry about chemicals, but do consider dust and molds.

SOLUTIONS

Substitutes for carpets include hardwood flooring, ceramic tile flooring or natural linoleum installed with nontoxic adhesives and wool and cotton or natural fiber carpets without stain-resistant chemicals.

If you have a new carpet (less than five years old) already in place, use a vapor-block sealant (liquid Carpet-Guard by AFM). If you purchase chemical-based new carpet, ventilate the room for 48 to 72 hours after installation and leave the premises. Also, let the carpet rest unrolled in a well-ventilated area for a day or so before installation. Look for CRI's "green labels" on carpeting that meets low VOC emission standards.

If you clean your carpet with a water-based cleaner, make sure it completely dries out to prevent mold from forming. Prevent conditions which foster mold by vacuuming often and keeping wet shoes or boots away from carpets, as they bring mold and moisture from outdoors.

Good News

The Carpet and Rug Institute, a trade organization to which 95 percent of all carpet manufacturers in the United States belong, has initiated the Indoor Air Quality Testing Program. Companies voluntarily participate in the program and sign a written agreement with CRI. If the tested carpet does not exceed established emission levels, it will be identified with the program label. If the level is too high, the manufacturer is requested to make formulation changes in the carpeting solution. The Carpet and Rug Institute information number is 1-800-882-8846.

A multitude of manufacturers are working to reduce emissions from their products by producing nonsynthetic carpets with natural stain resistors and low-toxicity adhesives. There are two kinds of safer carpet being manufactured. One is made from natural fibers, and the other from recycled or low-emission synthetic fibers (nylon faced with vinyl backing). Both promise reduced emission of VOC's.

State governments are addressing the toxic carpet problem. The State of Vermont decided not to purchase carpets that contain 4-PC and Dade County, Florida (including Miami) has eliminated carpets from schools. In addition, the New York attorney general has recommended that new carpeting carry warning labels about possible negative health effects, especially for children and pregnant women.

FOR MORE INFORMATION

Collins and Aikman low emission carpet (404) 259-9711, Georgia

Consumer Product Safety Commission's Carpet Hotline 1-800-638-2772

"Decors 4 U," Sutherlin Carpet Mill, LaHabra, California

Forbo Plain Linoleum Catalogue, Bangor Cork Company, Pen Argyl, Pennsylvania

Hendricksen Naturlich natural carpet (707) 829-3959, California

"Indoor Air Quality and New Carpet: What You Should Know," EPA 1-800-438-4318

TSCA Information Service (202) 554-1404

SYNTHETIC CARPET (Nylon & Olefin) INGREDIENTS:*

Ethylbenzene

Formaldehyde

Methacrylic acid

Methyl methacrylate

Low molecular weight acrylic
oligomers

Tetrachloroethylene

Toluene

Xylenes

4-phenylcyclohexene

Acetonitrile

Azulene

Benzene

Biphenyl

2-butyloctanol-1

Cyclopentadiene-ethenul-2-
ethylene

1,3,5,-cycloheptatriene

1-chloronaphthalene

Diphenyl ether

Dodecane

1,4-dihydroxyacenophthene

Ethylxylene

1-ethyl-3-methylbenzene

Hexadecanol

Hexamethylene triamine

1-H-indene

1-methylnaphthalene

2-methylnaphthalene

1-methyl-3-propylbenzene

2-methyl-4-tridecane

5-methyltridecane

Octadecenyl amine (oleylamine)

Oxarium

Polyacrylates (low molecular
weights)

1-phenylcyclopentanol

2-propylheptanol

Phtalic esters

Styrene

1,2,3-trimethylbenzene

1,2,4-trimethylbenzene

Tetradecane

2,3,7-trimethyldecane

Undecane,2,6,-dimethyl

*Excerpted from Hendricksen Naturlich flooring brochure

PAINT

DESCRIPTION

PAINT IN ITSELF can be hazardous, but associated products such as strippers and thinners can also cause sickness and death. A doctor at the Medical College of Wisconsin told the story of a retired executive who decided to strip a wooden chest of drawers. He applied a paint and varnish remover containing the common ingredient methylene chloride. After working on the chest for three hours he took a break, and after an hour suffered a heart attack. He survived, but two weeks later, he went back to stripping the chest only to have another heart attack, which he survived.

Six months later he felt well enough to attack the chest again, and after two hours of stripping he again had a heart attack. This time he didn't survive. It is surmised that the paint stripper fumes triggered the heart attacks.

Paint is a compound material consisting basically of a solid pigment, ground and suspended in a liquid medium such as water or oil. Today most oil paints are made with synthetic alkyd and epoxy resins and white spirit (a petroleum product that replaced turpentine as a thinner). More recent nondrip paints contain polyurethane. Urethane varnish and latex paint may contain insecticides and fungicides that off-gas indefinitely. Epoxy paints and varnishes contain synthetic resins and phenols that are possibly carcinogenic and have been banned in many countries.

Warning labels on paint which state "This material can be

106

harmful or fatal if swallowed, cause skin and eye irritation, and vapor mist may be harmful if inhaled,'' should indicate that these substances are hazardous to your health. Oil-based paints and urethane coatings have more volatile organic compounds than latex paint, but all must be considered as contributors to health problems.

Lead paint has been banned in the United States since 1978, and its use reduced in other countries, such as Great Britain, but it continues to contaminate people, especially children. It is dangerous because when lead paint deteriorates, paint chips fall off, and they can be ingested by toddlers. These chips and lead dust from renovation attempts can not only be inhaled, but may end up on the floor and on the hands of children (see section on lead).

Harmful materials in paints, stains and finishes that are high in volatile organic compounds (discussed previously) can include ammonia, benzene, ethanol, formaldehyde, glycols, kerosene, lead, pentachlorophenol, phenol plastics, toluene, trichloroethylene, xylene and heavy metals with toxic emissions. All are threats to health. Symptoms from exposure to the chemicals and heavy metal emissions include eczema, hay fever, arthritis and depression, to name a few.

Heavy metals can represent a long-term risk to human health and the environment because they cannot be broken down; in fact, they can present a significant risk even in trace amounts. Although oil-based paints present the greatest risks, both oil-based and latex paints contain such heavy metals as mercury, lead and cadmium.

New paints are being manufactured by several companies using plant chemistry without harsh additives such as formaldehyde, fungicides or toxic heavy metals. Most conventional paints are made from petroleum derivatives as opposed to the safe paints that contain naturally occurring biodegradable raw materials that reduce or eliminate sensitive reactions. Many companies, such as those listed later in this section, have entered into this market.

Paint Ingredients

Ammonia	Phenol
Benzene	Plastics
Ethanol	Polyester
Formaldehyde	Polyurethane
Glycols	Toluene
Lead	Trichloroethylene
Pentachlorophenol	Xylene

STATISTICS

One man's sensitivity can benefit the rest of us. Seattle paint contractor John Pruitt started experiencing shortness of breath and rashes on his hands and arms. This developed into liver damage, and Pruitt was forced to retire from his contracting business. He asked other painters whether they experienced symptoms and found similar complaints. Pruitt investigated further and determined that the chemicals in paint and associated products caused his sensitivity. This motivated him to formulate a paint that is nontoxic, low in volatile organic compounds and environmentally safe, and that performs as well as paints containing harmful chemicals. This product is now being manufactured as Best Paints and the contractors who are using it no longer complain about paint fumes, light-headedness and headaches.

Michael Bender wrote in the Oct./Nov. 1993 issue of *Green Alternatives* magazine that VOC's are a growing national concern, especially in the Northeast and southern California, where EPA clean air standards are not being met. During the process of out-gassing, VOC's mix with other airborne compounds, both natural and artificial, contaminating the atmosphere. When exposed to sunlight, VOC's can react with nitrogen oxides to produce ground-level ozone, a cause of respiratory problems in humans. Industry sources estimate that paints contribute approximately two to three percent of the atmospheric VOC's in the United States today.

Commercial painters are a high-risk group for illness because they are constantly exposed to the products they work with. The World Health Organization released a study that found the incidence of cancer among painters to be 20 percent higher and of lung cancer 40 percent higher than that of the general population. The *London Observer* reported a painters' union survey found that 93 percent of workers suffered symptoms associated with paint-solvent poisoning. These symptoms include nausea, headaches, hallucinations, stomach disorders and chest and lung problems.

A Johns Hopkins University study has found over 300 toxic chemicals and 150 carcinogens as potentially present in paint, depending on the manufacturing process. In recent years, mercury was used in water-based (latex) paints both as a preservative and a pesticide. Mercury was banned from interior latex paints by the EPA in 1991 following a well-publicized case in which a Detroit child was reportedly poisoned by interior paint containing mercury.

You will be reading and hearing a great deal about low-VOC products from all major paint and coating manufacturers. Low VOC merely means that the manufacturers are changing the petroleum-based chemicals and hydrocarbons used in their products to circumvent the California law which lists those chemicals that are carcinogenic. It does not mean that the products are any more suitable for the chemically sensitive or environmentally aware. We question, and so will the EPA, whether those products are any safer because they are less aromatic and whether they will outgas at a much slower rate, therefore increasing the amount of time we are exposed to them.

John Pruitt has contributed a listing of two common toxic ingredients in paint and their associated health implications. These substances (aqua ammonia and ethylene glycol) have been removed from Best Paints.

Aqua ammonia's routes of exposure through inhalation may cause irritation to the mucous membranes of the respiratory tract. Contact with the skin can cause severe irritation, and ab-

AFM Enterprise catalogue of products for the chemically sensitive (909) 781-6861.

sorption through the skin may cause severe burns. If swallowed, this chemical is corrosive to the digestive tract, and as little as a teaspoonful can cause death. Overexposure can cause atrophy to the eyes, cataracts, retinal atrophy and dermatitis.

Ethylene glycol, if swallowed, can cause abdominal pain, nausea, vomiting, dizziness, drowsiness, malaise, blurring of vision, irritability, lumbar pain and central nervous system problems, including irregular eye movements. Constant exposure can cause convulsions, coma, cardiac failure and pulmonary edema, as well as kidney damage if large volumes are swallowed.

In the late stages of severe poisoning, facial muscles may become weak, hearing diminished and swallowing made difficult. Just inhaling these fumes can cause irritation of the nose and throat, headaches, nausea, vomiting, dizziness and irregular eye movements, especially if the material is heated and a mist vaporizes into the air. Chronic exposure can cause long-term liver and kidney damage.

DETECTION

If a surface was painted prior to 1978, suspect lead-based paint and have it tested by a qualified lab or purchase one of the easy-to-use lead stick testers. These work by rubbing the applicator on the surface in question. If the stick turns color, there is lead present. One inexpensive brand, Lead Zone by Enzone, 1-800-448-0535, is available at Kmart and Walmart stores.

Most commercial paint contains chemicals; however, almost all stop offgassing several months after application. Read labels on paint cans before purchasing, especially to determine low-VOC brands.

SOLUTIONS

To avoid paint contamination, use many of the natural paints being manufactured, which derive colors and scents from natural biodegradable plant and mineral ingredients such as plant oils, tree resins, beeswax, clay, chalk, essential oils and plant earth pigments. Determine which brands have the least chemical components and purchase those. Consider casein (milk-based) paint, which was probably one of the original forms of paint, or go back to using whitewash.

Use shellac, a pure resin, instead of polyurethane. It seals up to 80 percent of the fumes emitted by chemically treated building materials, such as particle board and plywood, or apply a nontoxic paint sealer (restricts offgassing) to existing painted surfaces. AFM manufactures such a sealer. Paint in the spring and leave windows open for several months when using commercial chemical-based paints in order to reduce toxic buildup of fumes.

Good News

In response to regulations and pressure from environmentalists, major paint manufacturers have started producing low-VOC products by reducing the amount of solvents in the mix. Most of these brands are equal to or better than chemical paints in cover ability, texture and consistency.

California, New Jersey, New York and Texas have enacted air quality legislation restricting the amount of VOC's or solvents that paints can release into the air. VOC-limiting legislation is pending in all other states.

FOR MORE INFORMATION

Contact natural paint companies:
AFM (909) 781-6861
Best Paints (206) 783-9938
Livos and Bio Shield (505) 438-3448

WATER

HEADLINES ILLUSTRATE THE growing drinking water problems associated with man-made and natural pollution. *U.S. News & World Report* states that Hanford, California (population 33,000) still has not rid its water of naturally occurring arsenic, though it first violated standards more than ten years ago.

Thirty-eight toxic chemicals were found in the water of a neighborhood in Jackson, New Jersey. Residents' symptoms included headaches, dizziness, dysentery, skin rashes and kidney cancer. The chemicals originated from a waste dump in which 100,000 gallons a day of various substances were poured into an unlined pit right over the water aquifer. In Woodstock, New York, water containing asbestos from old water pipes forced residents to not drink or cook with tap water.

A headline in *The New York Times*, July 29, 1993, announced that traces of *E. coli* bacteria showed up in water tests in two sections of Manhattan. Inspectors were baffled by the bacteria, which should have been killed by routine chlorination. This type of water contamination showed up in the Midwest also. *U.S. Water News* stated that an increase in the number of allergy cases in Wisconsin has been linked to the contamination of Milwaukee's water supply in the spring of 1993 by the parasite *Cryptosporidium*. This outbreak cost the city $54 million in clinical treatment, water utility expenses and lost wages.

The Wisconsin Department of Natural Resources has begun a study of the contamination problem by taking samples from 20 watersheds. Residents in Los Angeles, California, were told to boil water following the January 17, 1994, earthquake in order

112

to prevent a similar outbreak: chlorination units were inoperative owing to power outages.

U.S. News & World Report, July 29, 1991, also revealed that Butte, Montana, is getting the reputation as the city with the worst water in the Rockies. Its 35,000 residents have to boil their drinking water at the same time each year because of high levels of harmful microbes, such as giardia, which can cause intestinal ailments. The Butte Water Company claims they cannot borrow the $20 million needed to improve their water treatment facility. Estimates drawn from Centers for Disease Control data suggest that more than 900,000 people are sickened by waterborne disease and that as many as 900 of those individuals die as a result.

Agricultural areas also share the limelight when it comes to water contamination. In the Orlando area 250 to 300 well owners are receiving reverse osmosis units from the Florida Department of Environmental Protection. This is due to exceedingly high nitrate levels in their water because of runoff from citrus agricultural sites. In the city of Des Moines, Iowa, for a month after heavy rains caused farm fertilizer runoff, levels of nitrates were 50 percent above the acceptable limit.

DESCRIPTION

Our drinking water comes from two sources: groundwater and surface water. Groundwater comes from wells, springs and natural underground aquifers. It is purified as it passes through layers of sand and rock. Surface water originates from rain that is collected in reservoirs that serve municipalities. In order to kill bacteria and other dangerous disease-causing organisms that may accumulate in these water sources, authorities put new disinfectants in the water. Unfortunately, these toxic chemicals have now been shown to have some very unpleasant side effects. Recent reports now positively link some of these chemicals to major health problems in humans.

A long list of water contaminants* includes lead, which not only comes from industrial sources, but from pesticides, paint

* See end of this chapter for chart of water contaminants.

dust and lead solder as well as older lead pipes. Nitrates, metals, petroleum, volatile organic compounds, brine, synthetic organic compounds, fluorides, radioactive materials, arsenic, agricultural chemicals and pesticides are only a few elements you may be ingesting while enjoying that glass of water. Ralph Nader's Center for Study of Responsive Law found U.S. drinking water to contain more than 2,100 toxic chemicals.

Our municipal waterworks are doing their best to provide us with safe and reliable supplies of high-quality water, but they test for only about 30 chemicals and only about 50 of our nation's 60,000 public water systems use modern treatment technologies that can remove these chemicals, many of which cannot be tasted or seen. These chemicals are known to cause cancer or inflict damage to vital organs such as the kidneys, liver, brain and cardiovascular system. Reports of the existence of these toxins may be altered to prevent the necessity for costly modifications to water treatment plants. The federal government won a suit against officials of two Vermont local water systems who submitted false test results.

In recent years, more than four of every ten U.S. community water systems violated Safe Drinking Water Act standards, including more than 15,000 episodic or chronic violations of federal water quality standards for water provided to 28 million Americans during the same period. The EPA found 48 to 49 states failed to adequately enforce existing water potability regulations. Seven out of ten Americans drink chlorinated water, one in six drink water with excessive amounts of lead, and tap water may be responsible for one in three cases of gastrointestinal illness from microbes.

Chlorine, first added as a disinfectant in the early 1900's, was identified as a potential health hazard in 1974. Scientists discovered that chlorine reacts with organic material, such as decaying leaves, in water to produce hundreds of chemical by-products, several of which have proved in animal studies to be carcinogenic. One class of these by-products are the trihalomethanes (THM's).

Chlorine has been linked to pain and inflammation of the mouth, throat and stomach, erosion of mucous membranes, vomiting, circulatory collapse, confusion, delirium, coma, swelling of the throat, severe respiratory-tract irritation, pulmonary

Ground Water Contaminants

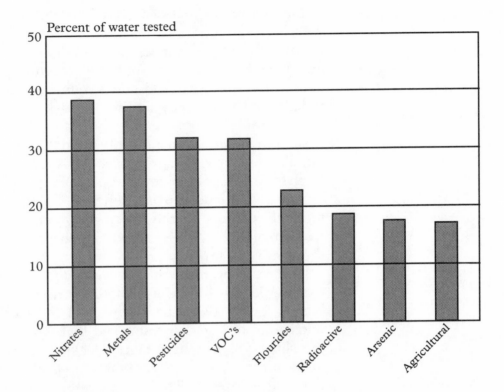

edema, skin eruptions, high blood pressure, anemia, diabetes, heart disease and gastrointestinal and urinary tract cancer. Chlorine affects the body through drinking water or breathing fumes from hot running water or showers.

Other water contaminants can also cause physical distress. Inside the mouth, stomach and bladder, nitrate can be transformed into compounds called nitrosamines, some of which act as potent carcinogens in rats. So far, research on health effects in humans are disturbingly incomplete. As reported in *U.S. News & World Report*, July, 1991, leading nitrate researcher William Lijinsky contends that nitrate pollution has contributed to the rise in cancer rates in the United States, but finds no conclusive evidence that nitrate in drinking water causes cancer entirely on its own. However, scientists are certain that nitrate in large doses can pose a threat to babies. In an infant's stomach, it is converted into a substance that keeps red blood cells from absorbing oxygen. In rare cases, this can cause blue baby syndrome, in which infants suffocate.

Radon can be ingested during bathing and dishwashing when the gas entrapped by water molecules is vaporized into the air. The EPA estimates that as many as 17 million people may have excessive levels of radon gas in their water. Preliminary studies in Maryland and Virginia suggest that drinking radon-filled water may double the risk of several soft tissue cancers.

Lead in water is a major problem, not only for city dwellers, but also for those using well water. A majority of contamination stems from old lead water pipes in homes and lead solder for pipes and faucets. Also, softened water can strip away the mineral coatings on the inside of water pipes, exposing the lead in pipes and solder and thereby causing leaching into the water stream.

Lead leaching from faucets was tested by the Environmental Quality Center at the University of North Carolina. Of 20 faucet brands tested, 19 leached more than the legal limit of half a microgram of lead. It is estimated that more than 17 percent of the nation's homes have faucets leaking high amounts of lead. Lead in drinking water, although rarely the sole cause of lead poisoning, can significantly increase total exposure to lead, particularly for infants who drink liquids made with water, such as formula. The EPA estimates that lead in drinking water can account for 20 percent or more of total exposure in young children. Some of this exposure occurs in schools and day care centers.

Fluoride, advertised as a beneficial ingredient, can actually be a chronic disabler. It is added to drinking water consumed by more than 130 million Americans. The EPA regulates fluoride at three levels: At 1 ppm it is considered helpful to prevent tooth decay; at 2 ppm, it can cause dental fluorosis, a condition indicated by stains on teeth that the EPA refers to as an "aesthetic" effect of consuming excess fluoride; at 4 ppm or more, it can cause skeletal fluorosis, a crippling human bone disorder, according to Joseph Harrison, technical director of the Water Quality Association.

The National Research Council indicated that dental fluorosis is the only condition likely to arise from consuming excess fluoride in drinking water. Until final conclusions are reached, however, be wary of ingesting this substance on a regular basis.

STATISTICS

At current drinking water safety standards, the risk of dying from cancer caused by arsenic is 21 in 1,000, or 200 times the EPA's acceptable limit of 1 in 10,000, according to University of California at Berkeley researchers. An estimated 350,000 people are being supplied with drinking water which exceeds the current arsenic standard, with at least 7,350 of them facing fatal cancer. About 30 million people are getting water which exceeds the 1 in 1,000 cancer risk.

The EPA says that as many as 40 million Americans have too much lead dissolved in their drinking water, and reports that 22 percent of large U.S. systems exceed the lead action level of 0.015 milligrams/liter (mg/L), mostly in the Northeast, Midwest and Northwest.

Kenneth Cantor and colleagues at the National Cancer Institute studied 3,000 people newly diagnosed with bladder cancer; they found that drinking chlorinated water may have doubled the risk of the illness. Also, the *American Journal of Public Health*, July 1, 1992, revealed that chlorinated drinking water is linked with at least 4,200 cases of bladder cancer each year and 6,500 cases of rectal cancer.

A study by the U.S. Public Health Service has found that exposure to THM's increases the risk of low birth weight in full-term pregnancies by up to one-third. That maximal increase was seen in women exposed to the chemicals at concentrations over 80 ppb. The current federal maximum is 100 ppb. The risk of birth defects was increased, and out of 81,055 births, 56 children were born with neural-tube defects. Eight were born to women exposed to THM's at concentrations over 80 ppb. Various chlorination by-products formed by toxic waste leaching into water also increased birth defects, including cleft palate and cleft lip, by up to three and a half times the normal rate.

Problems with drinking water are popping up all over the world. Portland, Oregon, supplemented its water from wells, which were closed recently after the discovery that five years ago, Boeing Company industrial solvents had leached into aquifers near the wells. Boeing has since begun cleanup operations, but the well problem still exists.

Groundwater contamination from agricultural chemicals can make drinking water a dangerous proposition. A study released by the National Center for Resource Innovations in Rosslyn, Virginia, has identified as high risk the areas from the coastal plains (Alabama, Georgia north to Chesapeake), the Corn Belt states, the Mississippi River Valley and the irrigated areas of the West.

Pesticides leaching into groundwater are not limited to agricultural areas. Nationwide, lawns cover 25 to 30 million acres, and suburbanites use up to two and a half times more pesticide per acre than do farmers to keep their lawns weed-free. These pesticides can leach into wells and runoff can enter conduits for reservoirs. An industrial leader in San Jose, California, discovered that one of its solvent-waste storage tanks had leaked, contaminating a well 2,000 feet away. This well fed a system that supplied 16,500 homes with water.

Studies show that chemicals such as chlorine, radon and arsenic may cause cancer and birth defects. One such study says the cancer risk from chlorine used to treat water could be greater than 1 in 10,000. Think of that next time you swim in a chlorinated pool or drink heavily chlorinated city water.

Most people know that arsenic is a poison, yet many are drinking it every day. The Natural Resources Defense Council cites a California study indicating that 2 ppb of arsenic in water poses a cancer risk. More than 350,000 people drink water with arsenic levels above the federal limit.

DETECTION

In order to find out if your water has unacceptable levels of contaminants, you can hire a local testing laboratory. Contact the EPA Safe Drinking Water Hotline 1-800-426-4791, for a listing of labs near you. Home self-test kits are available from catalogue companies, eco stores and major outlets such as Kmart and Walmart, but most of these are specific and only identify a limited number of pollutants. If you want to self-test for all of the contaminants in your water, contact National Testing Labs, 1-800-458-3330, for their mail-order kit.

Schools are becoming targets for ensuring pure water for children. The EPA recommends that schools take action if samples from any water fountain, water cooler, or other drinking water outlet show lead levels over 20 ppb. Approximately 10,000 schools in the United States obtain drinking water from their own wells, springs, or small reservoirs. They are required to perform the following monitoring of their water:

Parameter	Frequency
Coliform	One sample/quarter
Nitrate	Once (then as per state)
VOC (regulated)	Quarterly for one year
VOC (unregulated)	
surface	Quarterly for one year
groundwater	Once per entry point per well
all systems	Once every five years
Turbidity	Surface water systems only
Lead	Public notification as per regulations

Schools must test for lead in water if:

- The school system has lead pipes
- There are water coolers with lead-lined storage tanks/parts
- Pipes have lead solder
- Plumbing repairs have been made within the past five years and lead solder used
- Lead soldered pipes have soft or acidic water in them
- Pipes exist where water sits idle for extended periods.

SOLUTIONS

When treating for harmful contaminants such as trihalomethane disinfection by-products, consumers are cautioned to have their water tested to determine the specific problem; select equipment designed to reduce that particular contaminant; and follow the manufacturer's maintenance and operating instructions precisely.

Install proper point-of-use devices for your specific problem. (See chart at end of this chapter for type of equipment pertaining to pollutant reduction.) These water purification units differ as follows.

Carbon filters apply a water in/water out method so you get the same amount of pure as impure water going into the filter. There is no waiting for water. Carbon filters should be replaced every 6 to 12 months, depending on usage and contamination levels. There are different types of carbon filters for different applications. Activated carbon absorbs chlorine, pesticides, herbicides, radon, trihalomethanes and some organic chemicals. Activated carbon and Ecolyte (Sterling Springs brand) remove all of the above plus lead.

Amtek brand carbon/resin cartridges add mercury and cadmium to the list of substances removed. Carbon filters also come in portable sizes to use in travel in order to protect against, for example, heavily chlorinated hotel water. They are also sold as shower filters to prevent the inhalation of chlorine mist (as toxic if not more so than drinking chlorinated water).

Reverse osmosis systems remove up to 98 percent of dissolved solids in water including radon, pesticides, herbicides, nitrates, arsenic and fluoride. These units use about three gallons of water to make one gallon of pure water and, depending on the unit, can produce five to a hundred gallons per day. Carbon filters in the system should be replaced every six months and membrane filters every year or so depending on contamination and usage.

The *distillation process* removes most dissolved solids if it is equipped with a carbon filter. It is effective in eliminating microorganisms and removing particles such as rust and dirt. Distillers take as long as five hours to produce one gallon of water and require electricity to operate.

Ultraviolet devices are used to eliminate microbes and are added to carbon or reverse osmosis systems. They can exist as an integral part of the units or as an attachment.

Water softeners are a blessing to people who like soap bubbles and spot-free glasses. They reduce the mineral content of hard water by substituting sodium or potassium for minerals such as calcium, magnesium and iron. Since softeners can cut down on mineral buildup in pipes and appliances, they can cause leaching of any lead present in pipes; therefore, get good advice on the state of your plumbing before deciding on a water softener. Also consider potassium rather than salt as a softening agent. It is reportedly less harmful to the body.

If you have determined that you have lead plumbing, run the tap water for 60 seconds prior to usage to purge lines. Use this as a temporary measure until you can install a permanent filtration system or replace the plumbing. If you do opt for replacement, make sure the solder is lead-free.

Bottled water may or may not be safer than tap water. Before purchase, contact the manufacturer and ask for a copy of the water quality test to make sure of what you are drinking. One manufacturer, several years ago, was bottling Long Island, New York, tap water, contaminants and all. Today they process the water with a reverse osmosis system before bottling. Storage of bottles in warehouses under hot temperature conditions can lead to development of microbes in the water; again, ask the manufacturer how bottles are stored and what their average turn-around time is . . . the longer they sit the more the chance for bacterial growth.

Ozone is one of the most powerful natural germicides we have. In a study entitled "A Comparison of the Bactericidal Activity of Ozone and Chlorine," ozone was found to kill *E. coli* bacteria in less than one minute while chlorine took one to ten minutes to have the same effect.

Treating water with ozone is not new. Most European countries use it and over 20 U.S. cities are using it in some way. Ozone is used primarily in commercial or municipal systems. It is employed most commonly in residential applications to treat swimming pools, replacing chlorine. It does not irritate eyes, skin or mucous membranes, produce hazardous by-products like THM's and is not corrosive.

Good News

In 1976 Congress passed The Safe Drinking Water Act, which authorized the EPA to set standards for drinking water quality. These standards limit the amount of specific contaminants permitted in our water supply and are reviewed and revised periodically to reflect current health data and technological advance.

Amendments to the Safe Drinking Water Act being implemented in Oregon are dramatically affecting public water systems. Water systems are monitoring for many organic chemicals and other toxic substances for the first time. Some municipal systems have begun taking corrective action after discovering contamination. Water system managers are taking public notification more seriously and consumer awareness is increasing.

In 1986 Congress passed an amendment to the Safe Drinking Water Act known as the Lead Ban. The amendment requires that only lead-free pipe (not more than 8 percent lead) and solder (not more than 0.2 percent lead) be used in the installation or repair of any plumbing connected to a public water system supplying drinking water. In 1988 another amendment to the Safe Drinking Water Act was passed. The Lead Contamination Control Act focuses on lead in the drinking water of schools and day care centers. The EPA has posed radon limits for drinking water, but water companies have until 1996 to comply even though the technology for monitoring and removing radon is simple and inexpensive.

Local and state governments have been taking the initiative on water cleanups. The city of Des Moines, Iowa, is building a $4 million treatment plant to contend with high nitrate content in the drinking water. The city of Chicago is replacing old lead water service pipes. The completion date is 2013. Dade County, Florida, now prevents new businesses that use hazardous materials, such as dry cleaners and auto repair shops, from locating right over water well fields. Several towns north of Boston, Massachusetts are planning similar zoning laws.

On vending machines that distribute "purified" water, a California law requires the use of a monitoring device that automatically shuts the machine down when product water TDS (total dissolved solids) exceeds 10 ppm. In the absence of the device, the water must be tested each day and the machine shut down if TDS levels are too high.

Corporations also have increased consciousness about water

pollution. The 3M Company had reduced water pollution dramatically by recycling ammonia from a waste water facility into a base for liquid fertilizer. When Union Carbide Corporation discovered that one of their manufactured pesticides, aldicarb, was the cause of contaminated wells in Suffolk County, New York, it pulled the product and installed separate water purifying systems in 2,600 homes. Entrepreneurs are assisting too. One enterprising company installs activated carbon filters in hotel rooms on the contention that travelers will pay more for a room that has clean water. Let's hope more companies follow their lead so we can again have confidence that our tap water is drinkable.

One water filtration company, Sterling Springs, has initiated a television infomercial that not only promotes its product, but is designed to create an awareness about water pollution.

FOR MORE INFORMATION

International Ozone Association, 83 Oakwood Avenue, Norwalk, Connecticut 06850

NSF International (not-for-profit testing service), 3475 Plymouth Road, Ann Arbor, Michigan 48105

Water Quality Association Consumer Information (312) 369-1600, P.O. Box 606, Lisle, Illinois 60532

WATER CONTAMINANTS AND METHODS OF REMOVING THEM

	Activated Carbon	Reverse Osmosis	Sediment	Distiller
Arsenic		yes		yes
Barium		yes		yes
Benzene	yes	yes		yes
Cadmium		yes		yes
Chloride		yes		yes
Chlorine	yes	yes*		
Chromium		yes		yes
Copper		yes		yes
Cyanide		yes		yes
Fluoride		yes		yes
Herbicide	yes	yes		yes
Iron	yes	yes		yes
Lead	yes	yes		yes
Magnesium		yes		yes
Mercury		yes		yes
Nitrates		yes		yes
Odor	yes	yes*		yes*
PCB	yes	yes		yes
Pesticides	yes	yes		yes
Petroleum	yes	yes		yes
Radium		yes		yes
Rust		yes	yes	yes

*If carbon is part of system

	Activated Carbon	Reverse Osmosis	Sediment	Distiller
Sand		yes	yes	yes
Silver		yes		yes
Sodium		yes		yes
Sulfates		yes		yes
Sulfides		maybe		maybe
TTHM's	yes	yes*		yes
Zinc		yes		yes
Coliform				yes

APPENDIX A

COMPOUNDS FOUND IN HUMAN TISSUE SAMPLES (MORE THAN 100 CHEMICALS TESTED)

COMPOUND	PERCENT WITH TOXIN IN BODY FAT	SOURCE
Benzene	96	combustion
Butylbenzyl phthalate	69	VOC
Chlorobenzene	96	water
Chloroform	76	water
DDE	93	pesticide
DDT	55	pesticide
1,4-Dichlorobenzene	100	VOC
Dioxin	100	pesticide
Ethylbenzene	96	combustion
Ethylphenol	100	water
Heptachlor	67	pesticide
Styrene	100	VOC
Toluene	91	VOC
Xylene	100	VOC

Compiled by the EPA. National Adipose Tissue Survey of the Public Health Service.

Combustion: From part of the burning process

126

VOC: Volatile organic chemically unstable compounds commonly found in paint and solvents

Water: Synthetically produced toxins in water

Pesticide: Chemicals applied for pest control the residue of which is found in air and water

APPENDIX B
SYMPTOMS AND THEIR AGGRAVATING POLLUTANTS

SYMPTOMS	AGGRAVATING POLLUTANTS
Abortion, spontaneous	lead poisoning
Addiction	electromagnetic stress
Anemia	lead poisoning
Anxiety	electromagnetic stress
Arthritis	electromagnetic stress
	volatile organic gases
Aspergillosis	mold
Asthma	electromagnetic stress
	formaldehyde
	metal poisoning
	mold
	nitrogen dioxide
	pesticides
	respirable particles
	sulfur dioxide
	tobacco smoke
	volatile organic gases (heavy)

SYMPTOMS	AGGRAVATING POLLUTANTS
Back pain	electromagnetic stress
Birth defects	microwave radiation
Blood-brain barrier disturbance	microwave radiation
Blue baby syndrome	fluoride in water
Blurred vision	formaldehyde volatile organic gases
Breathing problems	sulfur dioxide
Bronchitis	VOC (plastics)
Burns on skin	microwave radiation
Calcium mishandling	microwave radiation
Cancer	asbestos (long term) chlorine in water electromagnetic stress fluoride in water formaldehyde nitrates in water pesticides radon respirable particles tobacco smoke trihalomethanes in water volatile organic gases
Cataracts	microwave radiation
Chronic viral syndrome	electromagnetic stress
Clammy skin	formaldehyde
Colds	electromagnetic stress formaldehyde mold respirable particles
Colic	lead poisoning
Collagen protein breakdown	fluoride

SYMPTOMS	AGGRAVATING POLLUTANTS
Coma	lead poisoning
Concentration difficulties	electromagnetic stress heavy metal poisoning lead poisoning volatile organic gases
Confusion	carbon monoxide
Constipation	electromagnetic stress
Convulsions	lead poisoning
Coordination problems	carbon monoxide lead poisoning volatile organic gases
Cough	formaldehyde mold volatile organic compounds
Croup	electromagnetic stress formaldehyde mold nitrogen dioxide pesticides respirable particles tobacco smoke volatile organic gases
Dental fluorosis	fluoride in water
Depression	electromagnetic stress formaldehyde lead poisoning mold volatile organic compounds
Dermatitis (acute)	volatile organic compounds
Diabetes	electromagnetic stress fluoride in water
Diarrhea	volatile organic compounds microoorganisms in water

SYMPTOMS	AGGRAVATING POLLUTANTS
Disorientation	formaldehyde
Dizziness	carbon monoxide
	formaldehyde
	microwave radiation
	mold
	volatile organic gases
Eating disorders	electromagnetic stress
Eczema	mold
	fluoride in water
Endocrine dysfunction	electromagnetic stress
	microwave radiation
	nitrogen dioxide
Eye irritations	mold
	pesticides
	sulfur dioxide
	tobacco smoke
	volatile organic gases
Fatigue	carbon monoxide
	electromagnetic stress
	formaldehyde
	microwave radiation
	mold
	volatile organic gases
Fertility reduction	fluoride in water
Fetal development impairment	lead poisoning
Fever	mold
	Formaldehyde
	volatile organic gases
Gastrointestinal problems	electromagnetic stress
	mold
	fluoride in water
	microorganisms in water
Genetic damage	microwave radiation

SYMPTOMS	AGGRAVATING POLLUTANTS
Glaucoma	electromagnetic stress
Grogginess	carbon monoxide
	electromagnetic stress
	mold
Growth impairment	lead poisoning
Headache	carbon monoxide
	fluoride in water
	formaldehyde
	heavy metal poisoning
	lead poisoning (high levels)
	microwave radiation
	mold
	tobacco smoke
	volatile organic gases
Heart problems	electromagnetic stress
	formaldehyde
	lead poisoning
	microwave radiation
	pesticides
	tobacco smoke
	volatile organic gases
Hepatitis	volatile organic compounds
High blood pressure	lead poisoning
Hormonal imbalance	fluoride
Hostility	electromagnetic stress
	formaldehyde
	lead poisoning
	volatile organic gases
Hyperactivity	lead poisoning
Hypertension	electromagnetic stress
Hypoglycemia	electromagnetic stress
	fluoride in water
Hypothyroidism	fluoride in water

SYMPTOMS	AGGRAVATING POLLUTANTS
Indigestion	electromagnetic stress mold
Infections	electromagnetic stress
Insomnia	electromagnetic stress formaldehyde lead poisoning
Itching	mold
Judgment impairment	microwave radiation
Kidney problems	chlorine in water fluoride in water lead poisoning pesticides volatile organic gases
Leukemia	microwave radiation
Liver damage	volatile organic gases
Low birth weight	trihalomethanes in water
Lymph node enlargement	volatile organic compounds
Mental development impairment	lead poisoning
Migraines	carbon monoxide formaldehyde tobacco smoke volatile organic gases
Mongolism	fluoride in water
Muscle ache/weakness	electromagnetic stress microwave radiation
Nausea	carbon monoxide formaldehyde tobacco smoke volatile organic gases
Nervous system damage	lead poisoning microwave radiation pesticides volatile organic gases

SYMPTOMS	AGGRAVATING POLLUTANTS
Nervousness	electromagnetic stress formaldehyde microwave radiation volatile organic gases
Nose irritation	respirable particles sulfur dioxide
Nosebleeds	formaldehyde
Numbness in fingers	volatile organic compounds
Obesity	electromagnetic stress
Physical development impairment	lead poisoning (child)
Psychosis	electromagnetic stress
Rash	formaldehyde insulation products volatile organic gases
Raynaud's disease	volatile organic gases
Restlessness	carbon monoxide electromagnetic stress lead poisoning
Shock symptoms	formaldehyde
Short temper	electromagnetic stress volatile organic gases
Sinus problems	formaldehyde metal poisoning mold pesticides tobacco smoke (heavy) volatile organic gases
Sneezing	mold
Spina bifida	trihalomethanes in mother's water
Strokes	lead poisoning

SYMPTOMS	AGGRAVATING POLLUTANTS
Temporomandibular joint (TMJ) syndrome	electromagnetic stress
Tiredness	carbon monoxide electromagnetic stress formaldehyde mold
Throat problems	formaldehyde mold nitrogen dioxide pesticides tobacco smoke volatile organic gases
Ulcers	electromagnetic stress
Vision problems	carbon monoxide electromagnetic stress
Weakness	volatile organic compounds
Wheezing	electromagnetic stress formaldehyde mold pesticides sulfur dioxide tobacco smoke volatile organic gases

APPENDIX C
POLLUTANTS AND THEIR EFFECTS

POLLUTANT	AGGRAVATED SYMPTOM
Asbestos	cancer
Carbon monoxide	confusion
	coordination problems
	fatigue
	grogginess
	headache
	migraines
	nausea
	restlessness
	tiredness
	vision problems
Electromagnetic stress	addiction
	anxiety
	arthritis
	asthma
	back pain
	blurred vision
	cancer
	chronic viral syndrome
	colds
	concentration difficulties
	constipation

POLLUTANT	AGGRAVATED SYMPTOM
	croup
	depression
	diabetes
	eating disorders
	eye irritations
	fatigue
	gastrointestinal problems
	glaucoma
	grogginess
	heart problems
	hostility
	hypertension
	hypoglycemia
	indigestion
	infections
	insomnia
	muscle aches
	nervousness
	obesity
	psychosis
	restlessness
	short temper
	TMJ
	tiredness
	ulcers
	vision problems
	wheezing
Formaldehyde	asthma
	blurred vision
	cancer
	clammy skin
	colds
	cough
	croup
	depression
	disorientation
	dizziness
	fatigue
	fever

POLLUTANT	AGGRAVATED SYMPTOM
	heart problems
	hostility
	headache
	insomnia
	migraines
	nausea
	nervousness
	nosebleeds
	rash
	shock symptoms
	sinus problems
	throat problems
	tiredness
	vomiting
	wheezing
Heavy metal poisoning	asthma
	concentration difficulties
	headache
	sinus problems
Lead poisoning	abortion, spontaneous
	anemia
	colic
	coma
	concentration difficulties
	convulsions
	coordination problems
	depression
	headache
	heart problems
	high blood pressure
	hostility
	hyperactivity
	insomnia
	kidney
	mental development impairment
	nervous system damage

POLLUTANT	AGGRAVATED SYMPTOM
	physical development impairment
	restlessness
	strokes
Microwave radiation	birth defects
	blood-brain barrier disturbance
	burns of skin
	calcium mishandling
	cataracts
	dizziness
	endocrine dysfunction
	fatigue
	genetic damage
	headache
	heart problems
	judgment impairment
	leukemia
	muscle ache/weakness
	nervous system damage
Mold	aspergillosis, allergic
	asthma
	colds
	cough
	croup
	depression
	dizziness
	eczema
	eye irritations
	fatigue
	grogginess
	gastrointestinal problems
	headache
	indigestion
	itching
	sinus problems
	sneezing
	throat problems
	tiredness

POLLUTANT	AGGRAVATED SYMPTOM
Nitrogen dioxide	asthma
	croup
	emphysema
	eye irritations
Passive cigarette smoke	asthma
	cancer
	croup
	eye irritations
	headache
	heart problems
	migraines
	sinus problems
	throat problems
Pesticides	asthma
	cancer
	croup
	eye irritations
	heart problems
	kidney problems
	nervous system damage
	sinus problems
	throat problems
	wheezing
Radon	cancer
Respirable particles	asthma
	cancer
	colds
	croup
Sulfur dioxide	asthma
	breathing problems
	eye irritation
	nose irritation
	respiratory irritation
	wheezing
Volatile organic gases	arthritis
	asthma
	bronchitis

POLLUTANT	AGGRAVATED SYMPTOM
	cancer
	concentration problems
	coordination problems
	cough
	croup
	depression
	dermatitis, acute
	diarrhea
	dizziness
	eye irritations
	fatigue
	fever
	headache
	heart problems
	hepatitis
	hostility
	kidney problems
	liver problems
	lymph node enlargement
	migraines
	nausea
	nervous system damage
	numbness in fingers
	rash
	Raynaud's disease
	short temper
	sinus problems
	throat problems
	weakness
	wheezing
Water pollutants	
chlorine	bladder cancer
	rectal cancer
chlorine by-products (trihalomethanes)	low birth weight
	spina bifida
fluoride	cancer
	collagen protein breakdown

POLLUTANT	AGGRAVATED SYMPTOM
	dental fluorosis
	diabetes
	eczema
	gastrointestinal problems
	headache
	hormonal imbalance
	hypoglycemia
	hypothyroidism
	immune system problems
	kidney problems
	mongolism
	reduced fertility
microorganisms	diarrhea
	gastrointestinal problems
nitrates	bladder cancer
	blue baby syndrome
	mouth cancer
	stomach cancer
radon	lung cancer
	soft tissue cancer

APPENDIX D
WHERE TO FIND POLLUTANTS

ASBESTOS

Automobile brake pads and linings
backing on vinyl sheet flooring
ceiling tiles
cement roofing
cement sheet, millboard
clutch facings (auto)
door gaskets in furnaces, wood
 stoves, coal stoves
fireproof gloves
gaskets
hair dryers
insulation paper around furnaces,
 wood burning stoves
ironing board covers
patching and joint compounds for
 walls
resilient floor tiles
shingles and siding
soundproofing
steam pipes, boiler and furnace
 duct wraps
stove-top pads

CARBON MONOXIDE

Automobile exhausts (in attached
 garages)
down-drafting from wood stoves
 and fireplaces
gas stoves and water heaters
leaking chimneys and furnaces
tobacco smoke
unvented kerosene and gas heaters

ELECTROMAGNETIC STRESS

air conditioners
beepers
heating appliances
high tension power lines

cellular phones
clothes washers/dryers
coffeemakers
computer monitors
cooking appliances
dishwashers
electric blankets
electric devices
electric shavers
electric stoves
electronic games
fax machines
fuse/circuit boxes
garbage disposals
hair dryers

infrared lamps
microwave ovens
portable electric heaters
radar devices
radios/clock radios
refrigerators
remote control devices
stereos
toasters
TVs
vacuum cleaners
water heaters
waterbed heaters
wired smoke alarms

FORMALDEHYDE

adhesives
carpets
exterior strandboard
fiberboard (cabinets and fronts)
glue
paint

paneling
particleboard furniture
permanent press fabrics and clothes
preservatives (wood)
pressed wood products
UFFI foam insulation, old

LEAD

coffee urns
decorations
food packaging
gasoline
housewares
inks
lead-acid batteries
lead crystal ware

lead paint
lead paint dust from sanding
lead-soldered food cans
pottery glazes
power plant scrubbers
solder
toys
water pipes

MICROWAVE RADIATION

alarm systems
CB's

radar devices
radio communication systems

cellular phones
diathermy and other medical uses
electronic games
microwave ovens
pagers

remote control devices
satellite dishes
signal generators
walkie-talkies

MOLD

air conditioners
central hot air heating systems
clothes dryers vented indoors
damp basements/crawlspaces
foggy windows
greenhouse/sunroom
humidifiers
improperly insulated walls without
    vapor barrier (condensation)

improperly vented bathrooms/
    kitchens
inadequate combustion for flame-
    fired heating/cooking
    appliances
indoor humidity level over 50
    percent
leaky pipes
leaky roofs
wet cleaned carpet

NITROGEN DIOXIDE

automobile exhaust from attached
    garages
downdrafting from wood stoves
environmental tobacco smoke

gas stoves and water heaters
leaking chimneys and furnaces
unvented kerosene and gas heaters

PESTICIDES

aerial crop sprays
ant traps, mouse traps
bug sprays, sticks, powders, crys-
    tals, bombs, no-pest strips
fruit tree sprays

fungicides
lawn sprays
rodent killers
termiticides
weed killers

RADON

in air inside buildings
in soil around and under buildings

in water

RESPIRABLE PARTICLES

fireplaces
kerosene heaters

tobacco smoke
wood stoves

SULFUR DIOXIDE

automobile exhausts from attached
   garages
down-drafting from wood stoves
environmental tobacco smoke

gas stoves and water heaters
leaking chimneys and furnaces
unvented kerosene and gas heaters

TOBACCO SMOKE

around smokers

VOLATILE ORGANIC COMPOUNDS

adhesives
aerosol sprays
air fresheners
antimold wallpaper adhesives
automobile products
carpets
cleansers and disinfectants
copy machine fluids
dry cleaning fluids
finishes
foam upholstery
hobby glues, paints, solvents
moth repellents
paint

paint strippers
particleboard furniture
permanent press treatments
plastics (soft)
polyester/cotton blend fabrics
printing ink (unless soy-based)
soft plastic shower curtains
soft plastic upholstery
solvents
stain-resistant carpet treatments
stored fuels
synthetic carpeting
washable wallpaper
wood preservatives

WATER POLLUTANTS

from acid rain
from agricultural runoff
from city water sources and
   reservoirs

from industrial pollutants into
   water sources
from toxic spills or dump runoff
from underground wells

BIBLIOGRAPHY

"A Breath of Fresh Air for Your Home," Honeywell, Inc., 1985 Douglas Dr. N., Golden Valley, MN 55422

"A Guide to Carpet and Your Indoor Environment," The Carpet and Rug Institute, 1992, P.O. Box 2048, Dalton, GA 30722-2048

Alexander, Syke, "Your Home May Be Making You Ill," *Earth and Star*, Dec/Jan 1992

"Annals of Radiation," *The New Yorker*, Dec. 7, 1992

"Are Your Homes Toxic?" *Builder Magazine*, Dec. 1992

Banks, Douglas, "Energy-Crafted Home Are Friendly to Natural Resources," *Home Daily Hampshire Gazette*, Oct. 2, 1992

Banta, John, "Nontoxic Termite Control," *Healthful Hardware*, 1992

Banta, John, "Using Air Filtration & Purification to Improve Indoor Air Quality," *Healthful Hardware*, 1992

Bender, Michael, "Paint," *Green Alternatives*, Oct./Nov. 1993

Between the Lines, "Too Much Lead in Water," *New Life Magazine*, March/April 1993

Binsacca, Richard, David A. Jones, "Building Your Own Greenhouse," *Builder Magazine*, July 1991

Bodanis, David, "The Secret House," Simon & Schuster, 1986

"Can Your House Make You Sick?" *Popular Science*, July 1992

"Checklist for Environmentally Sustainable Design and Construction," *Environmental Building News*, Sept./Oct. 1992

Clean Technologies, "Removing Volatile Organics," *In Business Magazine*, Jan./Feb. 1993

"Consumer Guide for Room Air Cleaners," Association of Home Appliance Manufacturers, 1990

Dadd, Debra Lynn, "Nontoxic, Natural & Earthwise," St. Martin's Press, 1990

Dadd, Debra Lynn, "Put Your Foot Down to Toxic Carpets," *Earth Star*, Feb/March 1993

"Decontaminate Your Ductwork," *Rodale's Allergy Relief*, Vol. 1, No. 9, Nov. 1991

Decors 4 U, Manufacturer's Brochure, Sutherline Carpet Mill, 450 Exeter Circle, LaHabra, CA 90631

"Do You Know What Is in the Air in Your Home?" Berner Air Products, P.O. Box 5410, New Castle, PA 16105

Dugleby, John, "Radon Alert: Is Your Home At Risk?" *Home Magazine*, Nov. 1992

Dust Free Air Purifier Catalogue, P.O. Box 519, Royse City, TX 75189-0519

Eight-Penny News, "OSHA May Regulate Work-Site Lead Exposure," *Journal of Light Construction*, Feb. 1993

Executive Report, "Contaminant Alert," *Water Technology Magazine*, Jan. 1993

"Finally an Air Cleaner Doctors Can Recommend," Austin Indoor Health Report, Austin Co. c/o Aquarius Health Shop, 7220 Porter Rd., Niagara Falls, NY 04304

"For Cleaner Indoor Air," NeoLife Catalogue, Fremont, CA

"For Every Breath You Take," VAnEE, Box 582416, Minneapolis, MN 55458-2416

Forbo Plain Linoleum Catalogue, Bangor Cork Co., Inc., Wm. & D. Sts., Pen Argyll, PA 18072

Ford, Dr. Joseph Scott Ph.D, P.E., "Comfort Management in Energy Efficient Homes," Engineering Development Inc., 4850 Northpark Dr., Colorado Springs, CO 80918

"Getting The Lead Out of Your Water," *Better Homes and Gardens*, May 1992

Gilman, Diane, "Saying Yes to Environmental Sanity," *In Context*, Fall 1992

Greeley, Alexandra, "Getting the Lead Out of Just About Everything," *FDA Consumer*, Jully/August 1991

Heins, Kathleen M., "Get Rid of Flu With Cleaner Air," *Health*, 1993

Hellmich, Nanci, "Experts Urge Lead Tests for Household Taps," *USA Today*, Jan. 19, 1993

Hendrickson Naturlich Carpet Catalogue, 6761 Sebastopol Ave., Suite 7, Sebastopol, CA 95472-3805

Hoffman, Ronald L., M.D., "Chronic Fatigue Syndrome Update," *New Life Magazine*, Mar./April 1993

"Indoor Air Quality Program for Carpet," Carpet and Rug Institute 1-800-882-8846

Introduction to Baubiologie, Institute for Baubiologie, Box 387, Clearwater, FL 34615

Jacobs, Robert L. M.D., Charles P. Andrews, M.D., Frank O. Jacobs, BS, "Hypersensitivity Pneumonitis Treated with an Electrostatic Dust Filter," *Annals of Internal Medicine*, Vol. 110, No. 2, Jan. 15, 1989

Jones, David, "Paint Primer," *Builder Magazine*, Feb. 1993

Jones, David, "Are Your Homes Toxic?" *Builder*, Dec. 1992

Levin, Hal, "ASTM Symposium on Bioaerosols," *Indoor Air Quality Update*, Aug. 1989

Lippert, Joan," Improving Indoor Air," *US Air*, May 1990

"Low-Down on High Efficiency Furnaces, The," *Home*, Feb. 1993

Meyerowitz, Steve, "Water Pollution Purification," The Sprout House, 1983

Nisson, J.D., "Surprising Field Observations on Forced Air Distribution Systems," *Energy Design Update*, Jan. 1990

Panda Air Purifier Brochure, Quantum Electronics, 31 Graystone St. Warwick, RI 02886

Pearson, David, "The Natural House Book," Fireside, 1989

Product Catalogue, "For the Chemically Sensitive and Environmentally Aware," AFM Enterprises, 140 Stacey Drive, Riverside, CA 92507

"Public Water Suppliers Exceeding the Lead Action Level," *Water Systems News & Home Water Report*, Oct. 1992

"Putting Renewable Energy To Work in Buildings," Union of Concerned Scientists, Jan. 1993

"R Plus and How It Works," BASF, 5850 Cote de Liesse Rd., Town of Mt. Royal, Quebec, Canada H4T 1C1

"Relative pH Tolerance," *Water Technology Magazine*, March, 1993

Rees, Ann, "Chlorinated Water Linked to Cancer, Study Shows," *The Province*, July 2, 1992

Robb, Maribeth Murphy, "The True Cost of Hard Waters," *Woman's Day*, July 1991

Sachs, Jessica, "Do V.D.T.s Cause Miscarriage?" *New Woman*, Dec. 1991

"Safe Home Digest," Lloyd Publishing, 24 East Ave, New Canaan, CT 06840, 1993

Sanders, Bill, "Shoppers' Guide, Carpets," *Green Alternatives*, Oct./Nov. 1993

Schomer, Victoria, "Environmental Illness and Multiple Chemical Sensitivity," *Interior Concerns Newsletter*, Jan./Feb. 1993

Smith, James K., "Calm Your Customer's Lead Fears," *Water Technology Magazine*, March 1993

Spencer, Elizabeth, "The Great Indoors, Vanquishing VOCs," *Home Magazine*, Feb. 1993

"Sterling Spring Brings Lead Reduction Solution to Syracuse," *Sterling Springs Press Release*, April 1993

Swartwout, Dr. Glen, "Electromagnetic Pollution Solutions," AERAI Publishing, 1991

Tunley, Roul, "Is Your Water Safe?" *Readers Digest*, November 1986

Vandervort, Don, "Tip-Top Taps: Water Purifiers," *Home Magazine*, April 1993

"Ventilation—Before You Build," Dec International, Inc., P.O. Box 8050, Madison, WI 53708

"Ventilation for Acceptable Indoor Air Quality," American Society of Heating, Refrigerating and Air-Conditioning Engineers, Inc., 1990

"Why Mechanical Ventilation," Washington State Energy Code Program, 1322 Harrison Ave. NW, Olympia, WA 98507

Yakutchik, Maryalice, "Is My Electric Blanket Killing Me?" *USA Weekend*, Jan. 1, 1993

Washington and Beyond, "Lead-Based Paint Disclosures Are Now Mandatory," *Good Cents Magazine*, Jan./Feb. 1993

"What Are Your Choices?" Well-Maclain, A Marley Co., 1982

Alfred V. Zamm, M.D., "Why Your House House May Endanger Your Health," Simon & Schuster, 1980

US News and World Report, "Is Your Water Safe?" *US News & World Report*, July 29, 1991

The following EPA Publications can be received by calling the Environmental Protection Agency at (202) 260-2080 or the U.S. Dept. of Energy at (202) 586-9455:

U.S. Environmental Protection Agency, "A Guide to Indoor Air Quality," US Consumer Product Safety Commission, 1988

U.S. Department of Energy, "Heat Recovery Ventilation for Housing," Appropriate Technology Program, 1984

Energy Administration Clearinghouse, "Moisture and Home Energy Conservation," Michigan Dept. of Commerce

EPA, "How To Reduce Radon Levels In Your Home," U.S. Government Printing Office

"Keep the cold Air Out," New York State Energy Office

"Combustion Heating Systems" Considering Whether To Improve or Replace Them," National Appropriate Technology Assistance Service, U.S. Department of Energy, P.O. Box 2525, Butte, MT 59702-2525

"Combustion Appliances and Indoor Air Pollution," CPSC, EPA, American Lung Association

"Asbestos In Your Home," CPSC, EPA, American Lung Association

"Indoor Air Quality and New Carpet," EPA, March 1992

"A Home Buyer's Guide to Environmental Hazards," U.S. Environmental Protection Agency

"Biological Pollutants in Your Home," CPSC, American Lung Association

"A Citizen's Guide to Randon," EPA, May 1992

"How to Reduce Randon Levels in Your Home," EPA August 1992

INDEX